Living with
Bipolar Disorder

MCFARLAND HEALTH TOPICS SERIES

Living with Multiple Chemical Sensitivity: Narratives of Coping.
Gail McCormick. 2001

Graves' Disease: A Practical Guide.
Elaine A. Moore with Lisa Moore. 2001

Autoimmune Diseases and Their Environmental Triggers.
Elaine A. Moore. 2002

Hepatitis: Causes, Treatments and Resources.
Elaine A. Moore. 2006

Arthritis: A Patient's Guide.
Sharon E. Hohler. 2008

The Promise of Low Dose Naltrexone Therapy: Potential Benefits
in Cancer, Autoimmune, Neurological and Infectious Disorders.
Elaine A. Moore and Samantha Wilkinson. 2009

Living with HIV: A Patient's Guide.
Mark Cichocki, RN. 2009

Understanding Multiple Chemical Sensitivity:
Causes, Effects, Personal Experiences and Resources.
Els Valkenburg. 2010

Type 2 Diabetes: Social and Scientific Origins, Medical
Complications and Implications for Patients and Others.
Andrew Kagan, M.D. 2010

The Amphetamine Debate: The Use of Adderall,
Ritalin and Related Drugs for Behavior Modification,
Neuroenhancement and Anti-Aging Purposes.
Elaine A. Moore. 2011

CCSVI as the Cause of Multiple Sclerosis: The Science
Behind the Controversial Theory. Marie A. Rhodes. 2011

Coping with Post-Traumatic Stress Disorder: A Guide
for Families, 2d ed. Cheryl A. Roberts. 2011

Living with Insomnia: A Guide to Causes, Effects
and Management, with Personal Accounts.
Phyllis L. Brodsky and Allen Brodsky. 2011

Caregiver's Guide: Care for Yourself While You Care
for Your Loved Ones. Sharon E. Hohler. 2012

You and Your Doctor: A Guide to a Healing Relationship,
with Physicians' Insights. Tania Heller, M.D. 2012

Autogenic Training: A Mind-Body Approach to the
Treatment of Chronic Pain Syndrome and
Stress-Related Disorders, 2d ed. Micah R. Sadigh. 2012

Advances in Graves' Disease and
Other Hyperthyroid Disorders
Elaine A. Moore with Lisa Marie Moore. 2013

Cancer, Autism and Their Epigenetic Roots.
K. John Morrow, Jr.. 2014

Living with Bipolar Disorder: A Handbook for Patients
and Their Families. Karen R. Brock, M.D., 2014

Living with Bipolar Disorder

A Handbook for Patients and Their Families

KAREN R. BROCK, M.D.

McFARLAND HEALTH TOPICS

McFarland & Company, Inc., Publishers

Jefferson, North Carolina

Library of Congress Cataloguing-in-Publication Data

Brock, Karen R., 1953–
   Living with bipolar disorder : a handbook for patients and their
families / Karen R. Brock, M.D.
      p. cm. — (Mcfarland health topics)
   Includes bibliographical references and index.

   ISBN 978-0-7864-5865-3 (softcover : acid free paper) ∞
   ISBN 978-1-4766-1512-7 (ebook)

   1. Manic-depressive illness.   2. Manic-depressive illness—Diagnosis.
3. Manic-depressive illness—Treatment.   I. Title.
RC516.B76 2014
616.89'5—dc23   2014019895

British Library cataloguing data are available

On the cover: woman with multiple emotions © iStock/Thinkstock

Printed in the United States of America

*McFarland & Company, Inc., Publishers
   Box 611, Jefferson, North Carolina 28640
   www.mcfarlandpub.com*

To my beloved family member who works so hard
to manage bipolar disease and succeeds beautifully
in living a productive, full and meaningful life.

Table of Contents

Acknowledgments

If one person finds the strength to hold their head up and go forward without shame, if one father chooses not to ostracize his bipolar child, if one daughter forgives her bipolar mother, if one person survives the worst that bipolar disease can do, all because of what they have learned about bipolar disease in this book, then I have done my job in sharing my experiences with you.

—Dr. Sis

A huge thanks goes to my amazing junior high school and beyond friend who so generously shared her experiences with me while I was writing this book. Because she firmly believed this book was important and relevant to bipolar sufferers and the people who love and support them, she opened up to me in ways I could never have imagined. Despite psychotic episodes and suicide attempts, she managed to fight her way back every time and lives an important, successful, and meaningful life. My friend demonstrates in unique, brilliant and creative ways that you can be bipolar and highly functioning if you manage your disease properly. Thank you, Dr. Sis. You are an inspiration.

I began this journey 13 years ago when a friend, Helen Clark, had the guts to confront me about a family member she suspected was bipolar. Like many people too close to a situation to see it for what it is, I was in denial about what was happening. While it is often difficult to face the truth when it is something we don't want to accept or admit, I will forever be grateful that Helen had the courage to tell me—a doctor who presumably knew plenty about bipolar disease—what I didn't want but needed to hear. Thank you, Helen. You are one smart lady.

It didn't take long before I realized that I didn't have just one family member with bipolar disease, I had more. Without the experiences and personal insight my bipolar family members have given me throughout my life, I wouldn't be writing this book. Some of those experiences have been amazing, others difficult, and a few terrifying. Thank you for loving and supporting me, as I hope I have loved and supported you. It's not always been easy, but family is family.

Thank you, Gil. Who but a husband would insist I needed yet another project to tackle in my "retirement"? Thanks also to my poet friend Alyce Nadeau, who gently but persistently prodded me to keep writing, always insisting that the world needed yet another bipolar disease book. Last, but certainly not least, a special thanks goes out to all my bipolar friends, acquaintances, and former patients, as well as their family members, who shared their stories and also their suggestions about what they wanted to see discussed in this book.

Preface

Bipolar disorder is a biological brain disease with emotional symptoms that affects, on average, around 2.6 percent of Americans, according to the National Institute of Mental Health. The majority of these affected individuals are considered to have severe disease and barely half are adequately treated, with serious financial, personal, and job related consequences. Many of these individuals inherit a moody temperament and are often considered extremely sensitive, difficult, and volatile, or sometimes hyperactive, impulsive risk-takers. Sadly, their disease too often goes unrecognized and therefore undiagnosed.

In writing this book, I have assumed the reader has either been diagnosed with bipolar disease or is close to someone with the diagnosis and desires to learn more about the disease. The book is divided into three sections. The first section provides a historical context for the disease, gives basic facts about bipolar disease, discusses in detail how the diagnosis is made, introduces the spectrum concept of bipolar disease, outlines the genetics and inheritance of the disease, and targets specific issues that bipolar women face. The second section is about bipolar disease treatment and discusses drug therapy, the various talk therapy options, lifestyle management, and experimental and alternative treatments, including nutritional supplements. The last section is about the good and the bad symptoms and the abilities that come with being bipolar. The lives of prominent bipolar disease sufferers, both historical and current, are discussed so the reader can see how real people handled their disease, for better or for worse. I deal only with adult onset bipolar disease—childhood onset bipolar disease is not within the scope of this book.

Names and details of bipolar incidents have been altered to obscure the identity of the bipolar individuals listed with the exception of Dr. Sis, who has allowed me to relate her experiences accurately, although I have given her a pseudonym to protect her privacy. I use quotes throughout this book from Dr. Sis, from several excellent memoirs by bipolar disease sufferers, and from historical bipolar disease sufferers to better describe the bipolar experience in

1

all its facets. There is no comparison between these incredibly descriptive quotes and my dry, academic definitions. I encourage you to read the memoirs from which these quotes have been taken, listed in the resource section at the end of this book.

The proper term for the disease is bipolar disorder but throughout the book I use the term "bipolar disease" to better reflect the seriousness of this illness as well as the concept of bipolar disease as a brain disease. Manic-depression is the older, more descriptive, term for bipolar disease, and can be used interchangeably with bipolar disorder/disease.

Introduction

"Is there bipolar disease in your family?" That simple question, voiced by a concerned and sympathetic psychiatrist, would forever change my life. I had referred a family member, whom I'll call "B," for evaluation after a friend kindly but firmly pointed out the unmistakable evidence of bipolar disease after I described the worrisome symptoms I had been told about and then experienced firsthand during my daily phone calls to B as we waited an interminably long two weeks for a psychiatric evaluation. B suspected multiple personalities because others had reported wild and outrageous behavior that had apparently occurred during black-out spells. Out-of-control angry outbursts had alienated nearly everyone in B's life, yet a few cared enough to eventually confront B about getting help. It was a combination of the memory lapses and friends insisting help was desperately needed that moved B to contact me. Normally B was a very controlled and highly functioning individual with strong boundaries, so this new behavior was confusing and very frightening. Since I was the only doctor in our extended family, B hoped I would know what to do and whom to call.

What B didn't recognize, and therefore didn't tell me about, were the catatonic depressions alternating with the frenzied, manic periods. In the daily phone calls to B prior to the psychiatric evaluation, I witnessed such a severe near-catatonic depression that I was seriously concerned about suicide. I didn't have all the details at that time about what had happened before B had called for help, but I suspected substance abuse, either for self-medication or as the cause of the black-outs and the severe depression. I decided not to ask because I didn't want to pry and I knew the psychiatrist would sort this all out in time. I had done what I had been asked to do—made the proper referral and then offered whatever support might be needed.

I'm not sure what diagnosis I was expecting, but bipolar disease certainly wasn't anywhere on my radar. To my knowledge, no one in my extended family was bipolar and we had no "crazy" ancestral skeletons in our closet other than a sketchy great-grandmother who had claimed to see ghosts, angels and other such visions. As a physician who has worked with bipolar patients in the past, I had a good working knowledge of the disease, although I had seen bipolars only at their sickest, when they were hospitalized or on their way to hospitalization. I obviously had no idea what a bipolar might look like before they "crashed and burned," as they limped through life dealing with their mood swings as best they could before diagnosis and treatment. Clearly, I had a lot to learn.

Isn't this the way it always is, though? What's right under our nose is often difficult to recognize and accept. I knew this or that family member was a bit too sensitive or immature and some were just plain difficult, but I suspect many people can say the same about their families. One family member was a former alcoholic who eventually stopped drinking and became a successful real estate entrepreneur. This was our family success story and something we were quite proud of. Excuses or explanations were always made for any aberrant behavior, including this family member's alcoholic binge drinking.

Don't all families make these same allowances for their personality quirks? This person was the baby of the family, was terribly spoiled, and has always been used to getting her way, or that person drank because he married the wrong person and that was his coping mechanism. Another person is stubborn (or moody, or smart, or bubbly) because aunt or uncle or grandma or grandpa so-and-so was just like that, and the apple doesn't fall far from the tree. Each individual's behavior and personality is interpreted as a part of the family history, but taken out of context some of these individuals may not seem so normal. When bipolar disease threads itself throughout your family, it is easy to lose your perspective on what is normal behavior and what is not.

Taken on the surface, my family history did not appear to be very impressive and to say a binge drinking, ghost-seeing, or overly sensitive or immature family member was mentally ill would appear to be a stretch. But the psychiatrist's question woke me up and forced me to see things as they really were and to stop making excuses. This was a smack-your-forehead, "a-ha" moment for me, when all my denial was stripped away and I could look at my extended family objectively and clinically. I realized that two of my family members were classically bipolar, with others somewhere on the bipolar spectrum. The mood swings were so obvious in the classic bipolars, including B—how had I not recognized this before? As difficult as it was for me to do, I had to answer, "Yes, there *is* bipolar disease in my family."

But first, I had more immediate concerns. Was B at risk for suicide? What did I need to do to keep B safe? When could treatment begin? How long would normal life be disrupted? Now that we had a diagnosis, all we needed was a therapeutic plan so we could get to work. Maybe we could turn this thing around quickly and get B back to normal. The sooner we could set the wheels of recovery in motion, the better. The right medication would set things right and restore personality and mood to what it once was. Right? *Right?*

How naïve I was! I truly had no idea how very sick B was. Things hadn't been normal for quite some time but I hadn't realized how bad they obviously were. Increasing instability had somehow been obscured during our brief visits, although there were signs that I would have paid more attention to, had B not been so much like another family member who, I suddenly realized, was also bipolar. I had explained away a good deal of B's increasingly eccentric behavior by telling myself that those two family members were just alike. As in fact, they actually were, only I didn't recognize why at the time.

It was only when I entered B's home that the seriousness of the mental illness became apparent. Normally organized and extremely neat, B was living in a shockingly disordered and chaotic environment. I packed up what I could so that B could live with me and get treatment locally, at the diagnosing psychiatrist's recommendation. It took a month to get an appointment with a psychiatrist near me, so the near-catatonic depression continued. The bipolar diagnosis was confirmed by the second psychiatrist and treatment finally began that unfortunately resulted in a full-blown psychotic episode six weeks later, causing a mad scramble to switch out medications and start all over again. That's how I found myself caring for a very mentally ill patient in my home, in addition to caring for the rest of my family and working. *How did I get in this situation?*

This beloved family member—so brilliant and creative and formerly so highly functioning—was terribly mentally ill. I could hardly wrap my mind around that truth. Suddenly the word "bipolar" leapt off the page and became a living, breathing entity in my home. It was the unwelcome houseguest that came to stay and refused to leave, the demon that tenaciously possessed my family member and needed to be exorcised but couldn't be budged. A three-week mental hospitalization was eventually needed for aggressive medical therapy and suicide prevention. It took nearly a year to get the disease under some semblance of control and another year for B to become reasonably functional again. Slowly but surely, though, B began to recover.

This disease had not come from the outside; it was as much a part of B as B's hair or eye color or height. It had lain dormant in B's genetic code since birth, waiting like a coiled snake to strike, and once it did, things were forever altered. I struggled with the feeling that the real B had been snatched away and replaced by an impostor. I held fast for a time to the belief that once the right medication or the correct dosage was discovered, the real B would finally emerge, but that never happened. Eventually I had to accept that the new B, forever altered, was here to stay, and somehow I had to find a way to make peace with that fact.

B's creativity and prodigious abilities were the bright, shiny side to this dark disease. I held fast to this one blessing as I armed myself with increased medical knowledge about bipolar disorder as well as my love and commitment toward B's recovery. I set out to discover a therapeutic pathway that would, I hoped, restore B's mental health without destroying the special gifts that came with the disease. As a physician, I wanted to learn everything I could about bipolar disease from the medical viewpoint. I spent weeks, months, and then years reading anything I could get my hands on, from medical articles and psychiatric textbooks to first-person accounts of bipolar experiences.

My family has been open about mental illness in our community because we want the stigma of mental illness to end. We want others to understand that people with bipolar disease can recover, reenter the world they temporarily left behind, and learn to control their disease rather than letting it control them, just as they can learn to control any physical disease they are diagnosed with. Yes, relapses can and do occur, but other diseases have their ups and downs as well. We want others to understand that bipolar disorder is a physical brain disease that presents with emotional symptoms. Diabetics need insulin, asthmatics need inhalers, and bipolars need their brain and mood stabilizing medications in exactly the same way. It is nothing to be ashamed of, yet shame and embarrassment are all too commonly associated with all types of mental illness.

When B was first diagnosed, someone advised me to be less open about the diagnosis because others would assume that my family was somehow "bad," but this is exactly why people need to be educated about mental illness. Maybe once they understand that mental illness is a disease of the brain, judgment and blame will cease to exist. I sometimes have the opportunity to teach about mental illness in my community and when I see the look of recognition on the face of someone in the audience who finally realizes that a problematic family member may actually be mentally ill, I know that one less person will continue to carry this stigma throughout their life. Perhaps their mentally ill family member will be treated with the understanding, compassion and respect they deserve rather than being feared or treated with anger or ostracized by the family.

I've used the knowledge I gathered through all of my research to help educate and support bipolars and their families in my community. This book is simply putting down on paper what I've been doing over lunch, in presentations, in the classroom, or in private homes for years. I have been given the opportunity to reach a larger community and I am grateful for the chance to share my knowledge with you. From the historical perspective of bipolar disease to brain chemistry, from medical diagnosis and treatment to wellness strategies, my hope is that I can give you the tools to first understand and then successfully manage and live with bipolar disease.

Chapter 1

How Did I Get Here?

Mrs. Mamone and the Divine Sculpture

"Mrs. Mamone?" At the sound of her name, a tiny middle-aged woman stood up, flanked by her husband and three grown sons, all wearing looks of anxiety and deep concern. Mrs. Mamone appeared calm yet slightly confused; she was accustomed to lavishing her family with attention so she didn't quite understand this role reversal. She allowed herself to be escorted to the door of the psychiatrist's office but she brushed off her men as she entered the room with quiet dignity and then closed the door behind her so her family could not follow her inside. Walking to the chair waiting for her in front of our intake team, she sat down and waited for what was coming. She had been here before.

Mrs. Mamone was neatly and modestly dressed. A large crucifix hung from her neck and rested against her bosom. As she leaned slightly forward in her seat, ready to begin the interview, she appeared friendly, pleasant, and cooperative. Her hands held a well-worn Polaroid photograph that she nervously fingered like a rosary, but now and then she paused to reach up and touch her crucifix. We glanced down at our scheduler's note: Acute Psychosis, family requests hospitalization. Was there some mistake? Surely Mrs. Mamone wasn't that patient.

The interview began, as always, with a few basic questions. Mrs. Mamone was a homemaker who had dutifully and happily raised her boys and cared for her husband. Even though her sons were grown and married, they lived nearby, so she had daily contact with them and their families and she found great fulfillment as the family matriarch. She was a deeply religious woman and a dedicated Catholic who found time from her domestic duties to attend Mass every day. After her father had died, she moved her mother into her home and had cared for her until her mother's death nearly a year earlier. Caring for her aging parents had filled the void after her sons had grown up and moved out of her home and she had especially enjoyed having her mother live with her. Yes, she had been sad when her mother died and she missed her constant presence for a time after her death. No, she wasn't lonely because she was never really alone, with the husband and sons and grandchildren in and out all the time. Her mother had lived a long and useful life and Mrs. Mamone knew she was in a better place. No, she didn't feel depressed. In fact, she felt better than she had felt in a long time.

We were confused. Why was Mrs. Mamone here? Nothing seemed to be wrong with this delightful woman, who seemed to have navigated her grief quite successfully. We decided to take a more direct approach and ask why her family felt she needed our consultation, but she seemed irritated and a little confused by our question. After some thought, she guessed her family might be worried about her because they thought she missed her mother, which of course was not true, she insisted. But as she said this, Mrs. Mamone began to finger the photograph in her hands more rapidly, turning it over and over, and touching her crucifix more often.

We asked her why her family would think this and she quickly replied that they sometimes caught her talking to her mother. She laughed as she explained how they thought she was just talking to thin air, so they assumed she missed her mother if she does something crazy like that. But, Mrs. Mamone insisted, her mother actually is there and she is the only one who can see and hear her, so of course she doesn't miss her because she is always with her. She did miss her, she explained, but then her mother came back and she's with her all the time and she can see her and talk to her anytime she wants to. She tries not to talk to her when her family is around because it upsets them but she sometimes gets excited and forgets.

And then Mrs. Mamone turned suddenly to the empty chair beside her and began talking excitedly in Italian to her mother. A few moments later she turned back to us and said that she had asked her mother to show herself to us but her mother had refused, insisting that she was there only for her sake and she didn't have to prove anything to anybody. That is so like my mother, Mrs. Mamone insisted, so doesn't that prove something?

We asked to see the photograph Mrs. Mamone had been holding through-out the interview, fully expecting to see a picture of her departed mother, but instead we found ourselves looking at a photograph of a popular downtown sculpture. When we asked about the significance of that sculpture, we were told that it had powers and had spoken to Mrs. Mamone when she had walked past it one day on the way to Mass. If she prayed to it every day on the way to and from Mass, it had told her, it would bring her mother back to her. She had decided to photograph the sculpture so she could pray to it even when she was at home. She had been faithful in her prayers and the sculpture had done exactly what it had promised to do. Although Mrs. Mamone didn't understand why the sculpture had more power than the Virgin Mary at her church, her mother's presence in her life was proof enough for her. Her prayers to the statue continued so that her mother's presence in her life would also continue.

We eventually discovered after further interview that Mrs. Mamone had been diagnosed with bipolar disorder in the past and had been well controlled for years on lithium. A visit to her family doctor six months before had revealed mild hypertension and she had been advised to lose a bit of weight and cut down on salt in her diet. When a friend had pointed out that lithium was a salt, she decided to eliminate that from her diet as well. The talking sculpture and eventually the appearance of her dead mother followed a few months later. We hospitalized Mrs. Mamone, much to her family's relief and to Mrs. Mamone's surprise. While she understood and accepted that she had made a mistake by going off her lithium, she adamantly defended the reality of her mother's presence and the power of the talking sculpture and insisted that her mother was with her in the hospital.

No one asked Mrs. Mamone to give up her delusion or hallucination. As the medical student assigned to her, I saw her every day of her hospitalization to monitor and document the status of her psychosis and delusion. As the lithium began to take effect she went from an unshakable belief in the physical presence of her mother at her side, and the power of the downtown sculpture, to some doubt, and finally to disbelief that she could ever have believed such a thing. Her psychosis resolved and she was quite embarrassed about the entire episode two weeks after she had been hospitalized. The tattered photograph was torn up and thrown away and grief counseling was begun to help Mrs. Mamone deal with the death of her mother—the second time around.

How Did I Get Here?

Mrs. Mamone appeared quite normal and functional while delusional and mildly psychotic, but given time, she would have deteriorated further. Her family had been through this experience in the past so they knew what lay ahead and were desperate to prevent a major psychotic breakdown. Fortunately for Mrs. Mamone and her family, she trusted them and agreed to see the psychiatrist and then agreed to hospitalization even though she didn't think anything was wrong with her. Bipolars commonly lose insight and judgment when they become hypomanic, manic, or psychotic, and they need trusted family and friends to intervene on their behalf. This should be worked out ahead of time so that when a situation arises where the bipolar sufferer needs help, everyone knows what to do and what is expected of them. Sometimes that is easier said than done, of course. But you can see in Mrs. Mamone's situation how well things can work out when a psychotic episode is caught early and treated effectively, so that recovery is rapid and a severe psychotic episode can be averted.

You may have had a similar experience to the one Mrs. Mamone had in that you didn't think anything was wrong with you but others were concerned about your behavior or your thinking. Perhaps you felt you were handling life just fine but friends and family felt you were in need of help. You may have trusted them and gotten the help they suggested, just as Mrs. Mamone did, or perhaps you sought help on your own. Sometimes paranoia and distrust can set in when your reality is questioned and you may have reacted with anger and refused to cooperate with those who wanted to help you. In extreme circumstances, help may come from the police or other authority figures in your community.

You may have had a lot of control over what happened to you, like Mrs. Mamone did, or others may have made decisions for you if you were incapable of making them for yourself. However you got the help you needed, I hope you will lay aside any anger and resentment you may have regarding how that help came about. It was a tough situation for everyone involved, I assure you. Be thankful that you are loved enough that someone wanted to rescue you. The alternative is much worse. If your family and friends abandoned you and didn't attempt to rescue you, try to understand that they fear mental illness because they don't understand it. Educate yourself first, get your disease under control, and then try to help them understand your disease.

Because Mrs. Mamone remembered every detail of her delusional, psychotic state, her reaction once she stabilized was "What was I thinking?!" You may remember everything, or you may remember very little if your bipolar mania was too high or your depression too low or your psychosis too severe. It's possible that you don't really want to remember such painful or embarrassing states of mind or actions. If you have little memory of what led you to your diagnosis, you may also be thinking, How did I get here? It's normal to feel confused and unsettled over the details of your bipolar attack. There is no need to rush to know everything you did or said when you were out of control. Sometimes it's better to look ahead and focus on healing and getting things under control than it is to examine the past. There will be plenty of time to deal with the past when you feel stronger. But if you feel you can't move ahead until you've looked backward, then by all means, find out whatever you need to know about your bipolar attack so you can begin to move forward.

What's important is that you got help, you are better, and you are now ready to face this illness and get on with your life. Your mind is clearer now and you are ready and able to take some control back, even if you might not have complete control over everything just yet. Recovery from a bipolar attack doesn't happen overnight. Be warned that your family and friends or boss and teachers will likely expect you to be back to normal long before you feel ready to rejoin the normal, functional world again. While it's great to have plenty of support, you can't allow your cheerleaders to push you faster than you need to go in recovery. There will be good days and there will be bad days. There will be great days and then there will be days that look for all the world like you have backslidden into illness again.

You have to work hard to keep your perspective and help your support team know where you are in your recovery and how they can support you properly as you recover. Baby steps and even backsliding are OK as long as your movement is generally in the forward direction. You may not be able to walk the dog on a windy day if you have a delusional fear of the wind blowing you away, but you can stand just outside the back door for a minute several times a day, then 2 minutes the next day, then 5, with your goal of eventually walking the dog on a windy day always in mind. Sometimes your progress may seem painfully slow but as long as it's progress, you are on the right track.

Your diagnosis and the details of your illness were probably explained to your family and perhaps to you, too, during your bipolar crisis, but you may have little or no memory of anything that was said to you at the time. Even if you remember everything that was said to you, you may not have been ready to accept your diagnosis or understand everything that was said to you. Now that your mind has cleared, you may have a lot of questions. How did I get diagnosed? What exactly did I do or say when I was extremely manic or depressed? Did I hurt anyone, either physically or emotionally? Do I need to apologize or make things right with anyone? What do my medications do? Do I really need to be on all of them, and for how long? Where do I go from here? How will this affect my future? You may look around you and everyone seems to be satisfied with your diagnosis and treatment while you seem to be the only one in the dark. How can you catch up? You may feel too timid to be assertive right now or you may even feel a bit intimidated by your psychiatrist or therapist or mental health team. I want to stress that they will never know you need help in getting up to speed on all of this missing information if you don't tell them what you need. They will be more than happy to backpedal for you, if you only ask them. Tell them you don't remember much of what happened, or you are confused about the little you do remember, and you want to go back to the beginning and find out why and how you were diagnosed. Let them know you have lots of questions now that you can think clearly again, and write those questions down as well as the answers they give you so that you won't forget them and can refer to your notes later.

If you encounter any resistance to this process, you may want to think about getting a new mental health team in the future if this sort of attitude continues, although I certainly wouldn't advise making any sudden changes in your treatment team (except in extreme circumstances) until you are quite stable. It's as important to have a supportive mental health team as it is to have supportive family and friends. While you can't change your family, you can change your friends—and sometimes you need to keep the friends who support you in your recovery and drop those who don't—but you have the right to choose a mental health professional you respect, like, and feel comfortable with.

Where Do I Go from Here?

Everyone's bipolar disease is different and everyone comes to their diagnosis by a different pathway. By the time many adults get their diagnosis, years of anguish, misdiagnosis, and medications tried and failed have come and gone. Guilt over things done or not done may have accumulated along with a string of lost jobs, damaged marriages or relationships, and ruined finances. Perhaps several suicide attempts or other risky behaviors have been luckily survived. There may be tremendous relief and an "a-ha!" feeling to having a diagnosis that finally "fits," but there may also be doubt or even periods of denial that come after the diagnosis. After all your experiences, particularly if you have been misdiagnosed in the past, you may have little trust left in the medical or mental health system. I want you to know that this is normal and expected. But stick with the diagnosis and treatment this time. You are finally on the right track.

While your mental health team will be able to answer questions pertaining to your specific situation, this book will give you a foundation of knowledge about bipolar disease in general. Educating yourself about your disease is the key to living your life successfully and keeping your disease under control. You can then approach your mental health team more confidently and build on this basic knowledge with the specific information they will be able to give you based on your particular situation. Unfortunately, not every bipolar is capable of a high level of functioning, so I can't promise you that. Not everyone is cut out to be a brilliant artist or novelist or musician or poet, bipolar or not. Some of you will struggle more than others because everyone's bipolar disease is different. If you are early in the diagnosis and treatment process, don't give up on yourself too soon. It takes time to recover from a major attack and you won't know what level of functioning you can achieve until you are down the road a bit. Success doesn't happen easily or overnight.

Some of the information in this book may seem depressing or even tragic but I refuse to sugarcoat the truth. However, I'm an optimistic person by nature who will assume that, with the right medication schedule, the right talk therapy, and a lot of hard work on your part, you can gain enough control over your bipolar disease to successfully manage your disease and live a full and meaningful life. But the only way you can learn how to live with this disease is to know it inside and out, and that includes the bad along with the good. The goal of this book is to show you how to function at the highest level possible given your specific circumstances. The fact that you are reading this book already shows that you are highly motivated to master your disease. My job is to show you how to stack the deck in your favor.

You may have had a bad attack. You may have been hospitalized. You may have been manic and done some crazy things or you may have been depressed and suicidal. That's over with now and you are on the road to recovery. Some of you are just entering that road while others are further along, but that doesn't really matter, because learning to live with bipolar disease will be a lifelong process and you'll get better at it as you go along. Will you have relapses? Probably— all chronic illnesses relapse. The more control you have over this illness, the less frequent and the less severe those relapses should be and that's a goal worth working toward. I've done my best to give you up-to-date and factual information as well as my own experience and expertise on bipolar disease along with examples taken from the experiences of a range of bipolar individuals. It will be up to you, however, to do the work on a daily basis and to use the information and tools you find in this book—along with the specific information given to you by your own mental health professionals regarding your unique manifestation of bipolar disease—to become as highly functioning as you are capable of being.

There is no magic formula here. You need a competent mental health professional or mental health team, a therapeutic drug regimen, some form of talk therapy, a stable daily routine including a good night's sleep, and solid support from family and friends. In a perfect world, right? When all is said and done, it comes down to you and what you are willing to do to be mentally healthy. You are the one who has to set up a daily routine and then stick to it. You are the one who has to take your pills on time, keep your prescriptions filled, and go to your doctor regularly to keep your prescriptions current. You are the one who has to keep your appointment with your psychiatrist or therapist or mental health team. While you may feel bipolar disease has taken over your life, you need to understand that by doing these things, you are the one in control—not your illness.

How badly do you want to be mentally healthy again? While you may never be the person you were before this disease struck, you can be a close approximation. You will be happier, more stable, more successful in your relationships and at work, and life will surely be easier than it was when your bipolar disease was untreated and out of control. But to do this, you have to make treating your bipolar disease a life-long priority. It may seem hard at first but once you get in the habit, it will become second nature.

Dr. Sis, a brilliant woman who is a musician and veterinarian and a friend of mine since eighth grade, suffered for years until she was eventually diagnosed with bipolar disease in middle age. She has graciously allowed me to use her factual information in this book, although I have changed her name to protect her privacy. She has survived numerous suicide attempts, been psychotic, lost everything she had worked for throughout her adult life three times, and has been hospitalized four times for psychiatric intervention. Yet today she is a highly functioning bipolar who has regained control over her illness and her life. She owns and operates a mobile veterinary clinic that allows her to make house calls to care for animals who are either too stressed, sick, or difficult to be seen in a traditional office setting. Although she chose veterinary medicine as her primary career path, she could have been a professional musician. I fondly remember her prodigy-level expertise and moving passion as she played the piano for me all those years ago. Today she plays classical violin and pursues this area of interest with the same dedication, focus and passion as she does her career. Listen to what she has to say to you about life after diagnosis and treatment, after many years of untreated or uncontrolled disease:

> There is joy out there. If I could find it again, then you can too. I can now see colors. I can hear music. I can kiss drooly dogs and feel the slime. I can smell horses. It is color, music and luscious smells that make you alive. I will tell you sometime just how low I have been and how far I have come back. I never expect to get well totally. I just expect to feel good (or feel anything for that matter) and stay alive, one hour at a time. One hour at a time.

Summary

1. Recovery from a bipolar attack takes time and patience.
2. Being confused about what happened or how you got diagnosed is normal—don't be afraid to ask questions when you are ready to know more.
3. You need a competent mental health team, talk therapy, medication, a stable daily routine including a good night's sleep, and solid support from family and friends in order to manage your bipolar disease.
4. You have no choice but to learn to manage your bipolar disease because nothing is going to make it go completely away.
5. It won't be easy managing your bipolar disease, but it's easier than living life as an undiagnosed and untreated bipolar.

6. Do you want to be a victim of a disease that controls you rather than you controlling the disease?
7. You must make managing your disease a life-long commitment and priority.
8. First you need to learn as much as you can about this disease that affects every aspect of your life.
9. This book will give you the tools to begin to educate yourself about bipolar disease and to help you begin to manage your disease.
10. What are you willing to do to be mentally healthy?

Chapter 2

A Historical Perspective

When I was growing up, society believed in a clear distinction between those who were mentally ill and those who weren't. My hometown, one of several large towns in South Carolina, had two prominent schizophrenics, one of whom attended my church sporadically, although his wife was a regular. The other was a woman I saw only downtown, particularly when there was a parade, where she could always be found out front in a sleeveless evening gown, even in the winter, leading the parade as our unofficial drum major. Both of these individuals were ever-so-interesting to my curious nature. I was delighted when the man from my church would answer rhetorical questions during the sermon; as a child, I never understood why the preacher would ask a question from the pulpit if he didn't expect an answer. I knew these psychotic individuals were operating outside the normal boundaries of adult behavior, but they approached the world in such a delightfully innocent and child-like manner that I couldn't understand why they made grown-ups so uncomfortable. There were adults in my life who made me uncomfortable and even a little afraid, but I never felt afraid or uncomfortable around these people.

Moon Pies

When I was older and working at a local downtown bank to put myself through college, I got to know the man from my church in a different way. He made his rounds every morning, handing out Moon Pies he had purchased in bulk and carried in a box to all the downtown businesses. If you're from the South, you can't help but love Moon Pies, and I was no exception. Since I was saving every penny I earned for college, this free snack was much appreciated. One day I noticed that as soon as this man left the bank, everyone threw their Moon Pies in the trash can. When I asked why, they mumbled and hemmed and hawed because no one wanted to say they thought the Moon Pies were dangerous because a mentally ill person had handled them. When I pointed out that the pies were safely sealed in their factory cellophane wrappers and that I had been eating them for weeks with no obvious harm, they remained unconvinced. I had known this gentle, generous, psychotic, yet reasonably functional man for most of my life, so I was shocked at the level of fear and paranoia I witnessed in the people I worked with. This is how I was introduced to the ugly stigma of mental illness.

One day, as this man was making his morning rounds, he came up to the bookkeeping department where I worked. He carried a brown paper bag in addition to his box of Moon Pies that day, so I asked him what he had in the bag. He told me he had found a gun in one of the alleys, and he pulled the gun out for me to see. Everyone around me panicked but I told him to put it back in the bag and he did. When I asked him what he was going to do with the gun he told me he was going to give it to someone who would know what to do about it. He visited the mayor and the police on his morning rounds, so I had no doubt he was going to hand it over to someone in authority. Unfortunately, he wasn't likely to alter his morning routine to do that first. Before I had a chance to convince him to take the gun to the police before he made any more deliveries, the police burst in and arrested him. I don't know which one of us was more stunned.

Someone in bookkeeping had called the police because they saw him pull the gun out of the bag. Yes, this was a bank, and the appearance of a gun in a bank is cause for alarm; but still, this was a gross overreaction and I get angry thinking about it, even today. This man ended up in our state mental hospital, where he stayed for 6 months because he was deemed violent and dangerous because of this incident, even though he wasn't either of those things. Somehow, "witnesses" claimed he had pulled a gun on everyone in the bookkeeping department, although I was the only one involved in the incident and I was never interviewed by the police. Again, I experienced firsthand the terrible stigma of mental illness.

Us Versus Them Mentality

Because society didn't understand mental illness at the time of this incident, people wanted mentally ill patients out of sight. Patients languished in mental hospitals for months and sometimes years even when they were capable of living out in the world; out of sight, out of mind was the feeling in the '50s, '60s and '70s when I was growing up, and before. It was lucky mentally ill individuals—like this man who went to my church or the downtown parade woman—who had a tolerant and understanding family who kept them at home.

During this same period, my husband's mother had a schizophrenic sister who had to be hospitalized a few times for worsening psychosis, but she spent most of her life at home with her parents. My husband and his siblings, and later my children, grew up with no stigma toward mental illness as a result of being raised around this aunt.

What society didn't understand at the time, but what a few families clearly did, was that mental illness isn't an "us versus them" situation. Anyone can suffer depression, given the right (or wrong) circumstances, and mania can be induced in anyone by certain drugs. People get anxious, have panic attacks, become obsessed, hoard, cut themselves, and suffer from addictions. There is a very fine line between normal and not-normal, and I'm not sure anyone can tell us exactly where to draw that line. Today, people are hospitalized if they are dangerous to themselves or others or if they are so unwell they are unable to care for themselves, not to hide them away from society. The focus today is on protecting the mentally ill, not on protecting society from the mentally ill, except in rare cases of criminal violence.

I learned about manic-depression about the same time this man was arrested and sent to our state mental health hospital. A woman I knew had been struggling to care for her elderly father, who had multiple health issues. This man seemed to have one health crisis after another; as soon as he got out of the hospital and back into his own home, something else would go wrong. One day, the woman was at work and she got yet another call that something had gone wrong with her father. She refused to go to the phone and had a "nervous breakdown" at work and had to be placed in a mental hospital for a month. Everyone was shocked at this breakdown because the woman had appeared as stable as they come, or so we thought. When she was released from the hospital, she told everyone that she had been diagnosed as manic-depressive and that her father was also manic-depressive and that was why caring for him was so difficult. What impressed me at the time was how normal she seemed in comparison to the gentle schizophrenics I had known all my life. Because I had never seen any mood swings in this woman I would have never guessed her diagnosis, although her son has been moody for as long as I have known him, so I suspect he's inherited the genes as well.

This all happened in the seventies, when not much was known about mood disorders, nor did society really want to know much about the topic. Hershman, in the preface to his book, *Manic Depression and Creativity*, comments that when he first began researching manic-depression during that era, there were so few books in the Yale library on the topic that he could check them all out and tuck them under one arm as he was leaving the library. He claims that the rise in the use of drugs in the youth of that era forced parents to confront the concept of who's normal and who isn't, as scores of normal but drug-addled youth were hospitalized with drug-induced mental illness (1). Suddenly mental problems came home to roost in suburbia and society couldn't ignore what had always been under its nose anyway.

Of course people have always suffered depression but managed to put on a happy face in public, suicides have always been with us but were covered up until recently, and the appearance of normalcy was maintained at all costs. There were drugs to treat depression and psychosis in the seventies, even if the side effects were a bit rough, and lithium was around to treat manic-depression. The stigma of mental illness was so strong, though, that most people didn't ask for help until they had no choice. Depression was seen as a personality flaw or the result of something that had gone terribly wrong in someone's life. The fault was outside oneself, not in one's inheritance. You couldn't risk tainting the family's good name or bloodline by showing any weakness of mind or character, so people often suffered alone until they simply couldn't function anymore.

Stigma toward mental illness is still prominent today, even if it has improved over the years. Today's society is more educated about mental illness than it was in the past and it understands that there is often a genetic component to these illnesses. Everyone knows there are abundant medications available to treat many of the psychiatric symptoms that occur with these mental illnesses, but for whatever reason, people still hesitate to actually ask for help. Primary care physicians are comfortable treating depression and sometimes screen for mood disorders and will make the proper psychiatric referral if needed, so a psychiatric visit isn't even necessary for the initial mental health evaluation. A serious disease like bipolar is best managed by mental health professionals, however. Today, it seems easier to admit to depression than to admit to being bipolar, but hopefully that stigma will continue to change. More and more celebrities and highly functioning people are admitting to being bipolar, and the more open these prominent people are about their mental illness, the weaker the stigma gets.

Ancient Bipolar Descriptions

Some of the earliest descriptions of bipolar disease come from the medical writings attributed to Hippocrates' medical school of the fifth and fourth centuries BC. Mental illness at the time was considered a manifestation of a physical brain dysfunction and if you can get past the main medical idea at the time—that good health required a balance of the four humors—you will see that this view of mental illness is quite modern. That's not to say that the average man in ancient Greece held this enlightened view. Most certainly did not.

The mentally ill, as well as those with epilepsy, were often shunned and sometimes removed from society and were a source of shame and embarrassment for their families. While the brain dysfunction view of mental illness served to lessen the stigma, at least among the educated, that stigma still remained quite strong in ancient Greek society. There were also some who continued to believe in supernatural causes to explain why certain people or families seemed prone to mental illness.

Aristotle, in the fourth century BC, also believed in the humors and considered the heart rather than the brain to be at fault in depression, or "melancholia." He also noted the tendency of some people to have repeated bouts of depression and he observed that some of them were quite gifted and highly functioning when not depressed. Among his examples were Plato and Socrates, and considering that Aristotle was Plato's student (and Plato was Socrates' student) he no doubt knew his teacher's moods extremely well. Even at that early time, the strong association between artistic temperament and "madness," particularly in poets, had been noted, although madness didn't necessarily mean psychosis but rather a heightened mood or state of mind we would call hypomania today. Priests as well as poets were thought to communicate with the gods through altered, divine states of mind. The connection between genius, the artistic personality, depression, and sometimes even psychosis was accepted then as it still is today.

There is written documentation dating back to the first century BC that mania and melancholia were a single disease with two different manifestations. But they weren't considered tightly associated until the second century AD when the cyclical nature of depression and mania was documented by Aretaeus of Cappadocia, who further characterized different degrees of mania, including hypomania and psychotic mania. The central idea of brain dysfunction as the cause for both depression and mania still held sway at that time and the famous medical writer Galen, also of the second century AD, introduced the idea that melancholia alone could be recurrent. His comments regarding mania suggested that it could be secondary to other diseases in addition to originating in the brain itself. Galen firmly believed in and expanded on the humoral theory of medicine, thus cementing the biologic basis of mental illness and placing such problems squarely in the hands of the physician for diagnosis and treatment, at least until the Middle Ages. Thus the medical model of mental illness dominated for a very long time, at least in educated circles.

The Dark Ages and Beyond

Unfortunately, as the Dark Ages commenced, all illness gradually fell under the cloak of the church and science took a backseat. Mental illness was blamed on the sufferer's perceived sins, possession by the devil, or even black magic. It would take until the beginning of the 17th century, during the Age of Enlightenment, for this religious influence to diminish and for true science to begin to return to the study of medicine, and mood disorders in particular. This shift of thinking resulted in more humane treatment of mental patients, replacing punishment or exorcism rituals. Eventually the era of Enlightenment transitioned into the Romantic movement toward the end of the 18th century and into the 19th century, where feeling trumped reason and logic. The Romantic movement was bipolar heaven; strong feelings and creativity were celebrated and encouraged and many bipolar artists, writers, and musicians thrived during this era.

Felix Platter published a description and classification of mental illness in 1602, but his description of the cyclical and recurrent nature of depressions and manias was unfortunately lost or forgotten and would need to be rediscovered. An interesting monograph regarding manic-depressive illness was published in 1759 by Andres Piquer, who was a physician to King Ferdinand VI of Spain. He diagnosed the king with what he called "melancholic-manic affect" (Goodwin and Jamison I:5) and clearly stated that while many medical books treated melancholy and mania as separate illnesses, he believed they were one illness, with the melancholia and mania linked together. He quoted Hippocrates and Aretaeus of Cappadocia to support his diagnosis, reintroducing the "one disease-two sides" idea once again. French psychiatric literature followed in time by describing the cyclical nature of depression followed by mania, or mania followed by depression, as "circular insanity" (Goodwin and Jamison I:5) and later, "double insanity" (Goodwin and Jamison I:7). Different degrees of mania began to be recognized during the 1880s as attention focused on the characterization of elevated mood states that didn't quite reach the heights of traditional mania. Hypomania (a mild form of mania) and cyclothymia (less extreme mood swings that don't end up in significant manias or depressions) were recognized, as were patients who were assumed to have only depressions but on closer observation were found to actually have mild hypomania rather than normal mood states when not depressed.

Kraepelin's Classification

Into this professional environment burst German psychiatrist Emil Kraepelin, who used his extensive clinical observations and impressive classification skills to make sense out of thousands of anecdotal, disconnected literature publications to bring order and continuity to the psychiatric field in Europe at that time. His colleagues quickly embraced his particular medical disease model of mental illness. The United States chose a different path, preferring psychoanalysis and psychological and social factors over brain dysfunction as the cause of mental illness. It has taken us a long time to catch up.

In 1899, Kraepelin formally defined the concept of mood disorder for the first time in the 6th edition of his psychiatric textbook. By 1913, the eighth edition of his textbook separated manic-depressive illness from dementia praecox—later termed schizophrenia—and placed nearly all of the known categories of depression at that time under the manic-depressive heading. Manic-depressive illness was described as cyclical, following a more benign course as compared to schizophrenia, and was associated with a family history of manic-depression. Kraepelin's data came from many years of careful and methodical observation of a great number of patients. Despite the fact that his classification was readily accepted clinically, it would take psychiatrists and researchers many additional years to study and confirm his conclusions. Kraepelin's classification remains our best working model for understanding mood disorders, even today.

After Kraepelin categorized manic-depression, there was always some criticism regarding his lumping all depressions within the cyclical manic-depression category. In 1957, German psychiatrist Karl Leonhard coined the term "bipolar" to describe patients with both depressions and manias and the term "monopolar" (now called unipolar) to describe patients who had recurrent depressions without associated manias. ("Bi-" means two, "mono-" means one, and the "poles" refer to the opposing mood states of depression and mania.) By doing so, he removed depressions he felt did not have any relationship to manias and placed them into their own distinct category. Leonhard also found that family history followed suit. Each group, whether manic-depressive or monopolar-depressive, was more likely to have a family history similar to their particular type of recurrent mood disorder, although sometimes there was overlap. A few studies subsequently confirmed that highly recurrent depressions were most likely a form of manic-depression, just as Kraepelin had suggested, supporting their inclusion under the manic-depression category.

The DSM Classification

The bipolar-unipolar classification of mood disorders was made official in the third version of the *Diagnostic and Statistic Manual of Mental Disorders* (*DSM*) in 1980, but, unfortunately, bipolar disorder was separated from all other mood disorders in the *DSM-IV*, thus uncoupling the unipolar-bipolar pairing and placing the emphasis on polarity rather than recurrence of either mania or depression. This would lead to years of classifying chronic, recurring depressions as non-bipolar, unipolar depression since the *DSM-IV* had no true classification category for patients with frequent, recurrent depressions. In other words, the term unipolar simply came to mean depressed patients without any history of mania or hypomania, considered by definition to be non-bipolar. Under this broad umbrella were single-episode depressions, highly recurrent depressions, and any other sort of depression that might occur. This is not what Leonhard intended when he developed the bipolar-unipolar classification.

Since the 1980s, bipolar-II has been recognized, where the bipolar depression may be severe enough to require hospitalization but the hypomania may be so mild that it escapes detection. Also, a significant number of recurrent depressions have been found to respond better to bipolar medications than to the usual antidepressants, strongly suggesting that these depressions are most likely undiagnosed bipolar-IIs. It has also been found that highly recurrent depressions are at least as common (if not more common) as traditional bipolar disease and share the same early age of onset, family history, recurrence of attacks and sensitivity to lithium. There are also rare cases of unipolar mania with no history of depression, although, as seen in bipolar-IIs, it's suspected that the depressions may be so mild as to go unrecognized, as they perhaps present as fatigue or a general lack of energy. So these cases most likely aren't purely unipolar, either. These individuals also demonstrate the same features of family history, lithium responsiveness, and early age of onset as traditional bipolar patients.

Manic-Depression Versus Bipolar Terminology

Leonhard may have coined the term bipolar in 1957, but the disorder was still being called manic-depression, by the public at least, for much longer. Many patients prefer the old manic-depression term purely on the grounds that it's so descriptive even a layperson knows exactly what the disease does. But the term comes with significant psychological baggage, conjuring up memories of great writers, actors, musicians, artists, and poets plagued by tremendous psychic suffering, madness and suicide. "Bipolar" is short and to the point and it fits the medical model of mental illness perfectly, although it might need a bit of explaining to the average layperson. Initially the bipolar term seemed clean and clinical with no attached baggage, although we've used it long enough now that anyone behaving outrageously or demonstrating a Jekyll and Hyde personality is in danger of being labeled bipolar. There seems to be some generational differences regarding which term is used. The older you are, the more you've been exposed to the term manic-depression in books, movies, and common usage, often with some stigma attached. The younger generation seems more likely to use the bipolar term almost exclusively and with less stigma. These are, however, different names for the very same disease.

Summary

1. While stigma toward mental illness still exists, society is better educated about the inherited mental illnesses, such as bipolar disease, leading us further away from the "us versus them" mentality.
2. The earliest descriptions of bipolar disease date back to Hippocrates, in the 5th and 4th centuries BC, when it was considered to be a physical brain disease.
3. "Madness" and the artistic temperament, particularly in poets, was recognized by the 4th century BC.
4. Aretaeus of Cappadocia first described the cyclical nature of mania and depression in the 2nd century AD.
5. The concept of mental illness as a brain disease was lost during the Dark Ages, when sin, the devil, or magic was thought to have influence over behavior and moods.
6. In 1759, Andres Piquer diagnosed the king of Spain with "melancholic-manic affect," quoting Hippocrates and Aretaeus of Cappadocia to support his diagnosis.
7. Kraepelin defined the concept of mood disorder in 1899, and by 1913 he had differentiated manic-depression from schizophrenia and placed all known categories of depression under the manic-depression category.
8. Karl Leonhard first used the word "bipolar" in 1957 to describe patients with both depressions and manias. He used the word "monopolar" for depressions without manias.
9. Chronic, recurrent depressions have remained outside the *DSM* bipolar classification.
10. Manic-depression and bipolar are two terms for the same disease.

Chapter 3

Bipolar Disease Basics

Wherever you have people, you have moods, and there will always be people who have moods in larger-than-life proportions. If those moods come and go on a regular basis, in cycles of minutes, hours, days, weeks, months, or even years, and those moods significantly disrupt an individual's life in some way, then that person most likely has a mood disorder. Kay Jamison describes having a mood disorder like this: "I long ago abandoned the notion of a life without storms, or a world without dry and killing seasons ... I am, by nature, too mercurial to be anything but deeply wary of the grave unnaturalness involved in any attempt to exert too much control over essentially uncontrollable forces" (*An Unquiet Mind* 215).

Mood disorders are surprisingly common and if you think back over all the people you've known in your lifetime, you will come up with a handful, likely more, of people who fit Jamison's description. Many, if not most, are undiagnosed and often remain that way throughout their lives and will continue to suffer from their mood disorders without adequate treatment. With treatment, they can lessen or sometimes break free of their mood cycles and the disruption their out-of-control moods cause in their lives. As Jamison says, "It is, after all, not just an illness, but something that affects every aspect of my life: my moods, my temperament, my work, and my reactions to almost everything that comes my way" (*An Unquiet Mind* 200).

We can organize feelings into three basic categories: emotions, moods, and temperament. An emotion is what a person feels in the moment. It may last from seconds to minutes, is triggered by a specific event, and can be quite intense. There is usually a physical reaction involved, such as a change in heart rate, blood pressure, skin temperature, or the size of the pupils in the eyes. Examples of emotions are a rush of love when gazing at your child, a flash of anger when someone cuts you off in traffic, or sexual excitement when you are with your love. Moods, on the other hand, last longer than emotions. Normally a mood may last for hours, but a person with a mood disorder may sustain a particular mood for weeks or even months. Moods tend to be less intense than emotions but can at times be quite intense, particularly in those with a mood disorder. These moods may be a reaction to a life event or they may arise spontaneously—the proverbial "getting up on the wrong side of the bed," for example. There is physical arousal present but it's less impressive than what is triggered during an emotion.

A temperament is a sustained mood state that serves as the underlying personality trait of an individual and it can last for decades or for life. A person with an even, calm temperament may occasionally fall into a bad or a particularly good mood, but their emotions will usually be calm and stable, for the most part. That's not to say these individuals can't get angry or have strong emotions. They certainly can if situations provoke or push them far enough, but their steady temperament usually protects them from extremes of moods and emotions. On the other hand, a moody (cyclothymic) temperament predisposes a person to exaggerated moods; therefore strong emotions and a depressed temperament predisposes to a depressed mood state and negative emotions. Thus a person's temperament predisposes her to certain mood states and, in turn, those mood states determine the emotions that person usually feels. Those individuals with cyclothymic and depressed temperaments are most likely to develop a mood disorder.

Normal Moods Versus a Mood Disorder

Since moods involve emotions and most people do not equate emotions, no matter how extreme, with illness, mood disorders frequently go undiagnosed. It is normal to have moods, of course. We all have good and bad days, but most of us do not have moods that go up and down on a regular, cyclical basis or find that our moods significantly impair our relationships or our daily functioning. Carrie Fisher describes having a mood disorder this way:

> Imagine having a mood system that functions essentially like the weather—independent of whatever's going on in your life. So the facts of your life remain the same, just the emotional fiction that you're responding to differs. It's like I'm not properly insulated—so all the bad and good ways that you and most of the people in adjacent neighborhoods and around the world feel—that pours directly into my system unchecked [113–14].

Fisher is saying that when you have a mood disorder, moods come and go mostly independent of life events although they are often blamed on external events or factors, which can seem to trigger moods. It is often difficult for people with a mood disorder to stop blaming life events as the source of their moods and to accept that the mood problem is already there, lying in wait for an excuse to manifest itself.

Why is it so hard to recognize mood disorders? We recognize sadness and depression or happiness and elation as proper moods, but we don't think of irritability, anger, sexual feelings, the urge to spend money, or surges of confidence as symptoms of mood states but rather as fleeting feelings we experience in the course of our day. Yet these feelings may be prolonged and even extreme when associated with certain mood states and can result in outrageous or dangerous behavior. Moodiness or excessive moods are often tolerated by the sufferer, as well as his or her family, friends and coworkers, despite the fact that they often make life difficult or unpleasant for everyone involved.

The moodiness of a person suffering from a mood disorder is usually seen as an aspect of their basic personality, not as a symptom of an illness that can be treated. The sufferer will invariably get the reputation of being hard to get along with, exhausting, argumentative, prickly, manipulative, self-centered, aggressively overconfident, inappropriately sexual, or, at best, overly sensitive, with feelings that are easily hurt. Not only do people with mood disorders overidentify with their emotions and mood states, seeing their "passionate" emotions as an integral part of who they are, others also define those people by their exaggerated mood states and learn to handle them with kid gloves or avoid them if possible.

Naturally, we do not see moods as symptoms of a disease but merely as a response to what is going on in our lives at the moment. Individuals with a mood disorder feel upset or depressed or nervous or irritable simply because the biochemistry in the mood areas of their brain shifted. Yet they believe they are upset because their husband or wife was mean to them, or they're depressed because they're in a dead-end job, or they're nervous because they have too much to do and too little time to do it, or they're irritable because they drank too much coffee or they didn't get enough sleep. A week or a month or two later, that same husband or wife is wonderful, the job is tolerable, that full schedule is invigorating, they are well rested, and absolutely nothing bothers them. Nothing changed in that time period except a shift in their mood.

For those without a mood disorder, life situations that precipitate uncomfortable moods and feelings motivate change in order for them to escape the unpleasant mood state that has occurred. An individual may decide to go to work an hour early to catch up on work, thereby relieving stress and increasing happiness on the job. Perhaps they decide to catch up on their sleep so they can decrease their daily caffeine intake and relieve some of their irritability, or they resolve the tension they have with their spouse. Mood states are often used as a warning sign, signaling that change is needed to improve the situation that brought on the uncomfortable mood state. Individuals with a mood disorder, however, are at the mercy of their mood states and they continue to blame external events as the source of their moods and usually do nothing to alter their situation. Even if they solve one problem, another will crop up to take its place and their mood state will remain stubbornly persistent, because their problems were never the cause of their mood state in the first place.

Of course, mood triggering life events can happen to those with or without mood disorders. But more often than not, getting off schedule, losing a night's sleep, or generic stress can bring on a mood swing in someone suffering from a mood disorder, without any attachment to a specific life event, although most of those people still manage to find something in their lives to pin a mood swing on. The real difference between those with mood disorders and those without, aside from a biochemical versus an external cause for a mood state, is how different types of individuals respond to their mood states and how much they identify with their moods. Those without a mood disorder are more likely to recognize that a life event or a stressful situation has precipitated their mood state. They don't necessarily see themselves as a suffering, martyred person when depressed or think they are so wonderful and special when they are feeling good that they will feel this way forever. They know that both bad and good moods are temporary. Mood disorder sufferers often wallow in the depths of depression, feeling so worthless and ineffectual that they don't or can't take any action to alter their mood state. When they are hypomanic or mildly manic, they feel as if this mood state is the manifestation of who they really are so they have no motivation to alter it. In other words, those with mood disorders become their moods, in a sense. When they are in a mood, they feel as if it will last forever and that it represents the essence of who they are. Those who don't suffer from a mood disorder recognize that mood states are fleeting. They enjoy feeling good while it lasts, they try to improve whatever bad mood they may find themselves in, but they always know they will eventually return to their baseline mood, which represents who they really are.

Most people with mood disorders see their behavior very differently than their friends and family do. While mood disorder sufferers blame external life events to explain the way they behave or feel, their friends and family insist that the person has always been moody and they can accurately predict how that person will react, regardless of whatever external life event might occur. Often, those close to the mood sufferer "walk on eggshells" in order to avoid a mood blowup, knowing that it doesn't take much to trigger a mood episode. I've experienced that myself. One family member has ruined more than a few dinners, vacations, and holiday celebrations by taking a random conversational comment personally or by getting upset when plans don't go as expected. The "quiet and peaceful life" an untreated family member insists is being lived is filled with veiled threats of suicide when this person is depressed and can be chaotic and dangerous when mania and psychosis take over, leaving a wake of destroyed family relationships in the path of extreme denial about having bipolar disease.

So how do you know if you have a mood disorder or just an eventful life? If your moods are extreme and wax and wane on a cyclical basis, then there's a biochemical cause at the root of your mood states, and biochemical mood swings equal mood disorder. It's easy to fall into the trap of always blaming something or somebody for your moods when actually your mood came first and you are simply looking for an excuse to blame the mood on. You make the very natural mistake of assuming that the origin of your mood came from outside of you rather than from within. Great husband, horrible husband, perfect job, disaster job—when you find yourself caught in these up-and-down mood states in a regular pattern, over and over again, you can suspect a mood disorder.

Don't fall in the trap of using external excuses, as tempting as it may be, to explain your internal biochemical moods if you recognize this back and forth pattern in yourself. Understand that the mood comes first and your brain naturally seeks to find an explanation for the reason you feel the way you do. Disconnecting your internal mood from external events may help you step back and wait out the mood so as not to act on impulse and destroy a relationship or act in ways you may later regret. If you are unaware or unconvinced of the cyclical nature of your moods, try keeping a mood diary for a few months. You can do this in diary, spreadsheet, or graph format, or even use the free iPhone app MoodPanda, which provides both diary and graph formats. If a pattern of cyclical mood swings exists, a mood record of this sort will reveal the trend to you.

Mood Disorders

You will sometimes see mood disorders referred to as affective disorders. Those terms are equivalent. A person's "affect" is how their mood appears to others, their facial expression or posture and body language, for example. The term "affective disorder" was originally used to describe the condition causing the "affect." For example, depression is an affective disorder causing an affect that might be described as a sad facial expression in a person who is sitting very still, slumped over with head hanging and with slow, deliberate body movements. The term "mood disorder" is used now instead of affective disorder because it best describes why someone has the affect they do—what's going on inside them to give them the facial expression or body posture they have.

There are two basic categories of mood disorder, Depressive Disorders and Bipolar Disorders, although the newly revised American Psychiatric Association's *DSM-V* has done away with the mood disorders classification entirely (65–114). Major Depressive Disorder was divided into two categories in the past: depression that occurs as a single episode and depression that recurs, but that distinction is gone in the new *DSM*. Highly recurrent depressions are felt by some experts to represent a subtype of bipolar disorder and were originally included in the bipolar category but are not distinguished in any way from single episode depressions currently. All types of depressions not involving obvious mania or hypomania are now included under the Depressive Disorder category, including Disruptive Mood Dysregulation Disorder (93–94), Persistent Depressant Disorder (Dysthymia) (97–99), Premenstrual Dysphoric Disorder (100–1), and depressions involving agitation, psychosis, a seasonal or peripartum pattern or onset, or have signs of, but don't quite meet, the criteria for hypomania or mania (107–14). Many of these disorders most likely lie somewhere on the bipolar spectrum.

Depression related to substance abuse, particularly alcohol abuse and chronic, long-term use of benzodiazepines, is included under the Depressive Disorders category (101–2). There is a high suicide rate associated with alcohol abuse, and while some may use alcohol as self-medication for a preexisting mood disorder, others have alcohol-induced depression that completely resolves once they are sober. It can be difficult to know if a mood disorder preceded the alcohol abuse or was caused by it. And because some of the mood stabilizers cannot be safely taken with alcohol due to the risk of liver toxicity, withdrawal from alcohol must occur before treatment begins. If the mood disorder improves or resolves after sobriety is achieved but before treatment has begun, alcohol was likely the original cause of the mood disorder. If withdrawal results in no improvement or even a worsening of the mood disorder, then treatment with mood stabilizers can safely begin, assuming liver function is normal. Withdrawal after long-term use of benzodiazepines can cause depression even if the withdrawal is gradual. While the depression usually improves in a few months, it occasionally can last up to a year.

Mood States in Bipolar Disease

The manic mood state involves an elevated mood approaching euphoria with grandiosity (delusions of grandeur). Carrie Fisher says, "When you're manic, every urge is like an edict from the Vatican.... Mania is, in effect, liquid confidence" (128). This feeling of grandiosity can lead to disastrous consequences. Mania begins as hypomania, which is a milder version of mania, and may be minimal enough not to disrupt the sufferer's life but can sometimes cause problems. Mild hypomania is often overlooked and therefore underreported, as many of its features, taken out of context, are not usually considered signs of mental illness. The hypomanic feels self-confident, happy, energetic, and in control, but the closer the hypomania approaches the level of mania, the more things begin to spin out of control. Terri Cheney describes the transition from hypomania to mania like this: "Happiness is fine, in it's season, but happiness out of season is a sure harbinger of doom.... It was just another checkpoint on the road to mania.... What felt like happy now might well be *too* happy in a minute—and we all knew where too happy could lead" (33).

The heightened mental abilities enjoyed in hypomania may first progress to scattered, rapid thoughts and then deteriorate to disjointed and bizarre thinking. The increased energy of hypomania transitions into sleepless nights and frantic, active days of nonstop activity. Rapid, fluent speech may turn into a nonstop stream-of-consciousness babble or constant writing. Irritability and paranoia may be present, igniting outbursts of anger if the emerging manic is blocked or thwarted in any way. Decision-making declines and judgment becomes extremely poor. Great sums of money may be spent during advanced hypomania or mania and physical risks may be taken that wouldn't ordinarily be considered, much less acted on, such as risky sexual behavior or reckless driving. In acute mania, delusions and psychosis with hallucinations may occur. When a individual is in an acute manic state, there is never any question they are mentally ill.

The depressed mood state involves a decrease in mood but also a decrease in energy, speed of speech, thought and activity level. Marya Hornbacher describes bipolar depression as "a painful hole yawning open in my chest. This old, familiar ache does not feel so much like sadness as it does like death, if death is blunt and heavy and topples into you, knocking you flat" (57). Some bipolars describe a general lack of feeling along with a dulling of mental capacities, including emotional expression, so it's not uncommon for a bipolar to deny feeling sad or even depressed—they simply don't feel anything at all. There is also a decreased interest in sex or any of the usual pleasures the sufferer normally enjoys, fostering a feeling of despair, pessimism, or worse, death. While the types of delusions or hallucinations typical to mania are not usually present in depression, there may be exaggerated concern over minor physical aches and pains so that fears about serious physical illness loom large in the depressed bipolar's mind, fostering a hypochondriacal delusional state. Irrational fears, obsessing over disturbing thoughts, and panic attacks are common. An overwhelming fatigue is often present and the depressed sufferer will often withdraw from society, including friends and family. Sleep and eating patterns will be severely disrupted, with the individual either eating and sleeping too much or too little. Suicidal thinking is common, as life seems too painful to continue. Since time seems to slow to a crawl, this mood state appears to last forever to those who are in its throes.

Pure mood states, where a mood is all hypomania/mania or all depression, rarely exist in reality and there is often a great deal of overlap as one mood state slowly morphs into another, flips back and forth rapidly, or swirls together in a constant state of change. I've heard the term "multipolarity" used to describe this concept of mood overlap, where one mood state may dominate but features of the other mood state are also present. For example, a person may be hypomanic and feel predominately euphoric but may also be extremely irritable, impatient and angry. When features of both mood states are present we define this as a mixed mood state, but in reality, most mood states are mixed, to varying degrees (Bauer, Simon, and Ludman). The fluidity of bipolar mood states makes the task of trying to classify such a complex and variable disease difficult and requires simplification that, in turn, leads to a predictably less-than-accurate definition of its categories. The concept of the bipolar spectrum has helped find a place for those clinical presentations that don't quite fit into the more common bipolar categories. The hypomanic/manic, depressed, and mixed mood states will be discussed in more detail in chapter 4, "Bipolar Disease Diagnosis."

Bipolar Disease Definition

"Manic depression is ... about blips and burps of madness, moments of absolute delusion, bliss, and irrational and dangerous choices made in order to heighten pleasure and excitement and to ensure a sense of control" (Behrman xviii). This is Andy Behrman's definition of bipolar disease, as he experienced it. He remained in hypomania with leaps into mania for several years before he began to develop the classic symptoms of bipolar-I, complete with severe depressions and manic psychosis. The classic definition of bipolar disease involves a change from one mood state, either depression or mania, to the other. For practical purposes we will consider bipolar disease an illness where the moods change from high to low but with considerable mixing of mood states during this transition between states. The mood states can be so extreme that normal functioning is impaired, and these mood state changes occur on a cyclical basis.

There are two main classifications of bipolar disease called bipolar-I and bipolar-II. In bipolar-I, the classic mood swings from mania to depression occur on a regular basis, sometimes with a period of normal mood between the two mood states. The timing varies for these mood shifts and some people may switch moods over several years while others may switch several times in a day. Bipolar-II is often mistaken for chronic, recurrent depression because the hypomanias are usually so subtle that the sufferer assumes he is feeling good only after emerging from a long and difficult depression. Bipolar-IIs may not respond to typical antidepressant medication. But they usually respond to bipolar medication, and that's why proper diagnosis is important for these individuals. There are other subtypes of bipolar disease which will be discussed later in the book, for bipolar appears to be a spectrum disorder where those who inherit the genes may range from having a moody temperament all the way to having full-blown bipolar-I disease. There is a lot of room between these two extremes for quite a stunning array of symptom manifestation.

When we mention the various mood states of bipolar disease, we will simplify the discussion by assuming that these mood states are pure. But keep in mind that in reality these states significantly overlap in daily life. The details of bipolar disease will vary from person to person—how high or how low each mood will go, the degree of mood overlap that occurs, the timing of the cycles, whether mania or depression will predominate, and if losing touch with reality (psychosis) or suicidal thinking will occur. While the basic characteristics of the disease remain the same, each person will have a unique manifestation of bipolar, as they would in any physical disease. We will discuss the specific details of bipolar disease in later chapters.

Bipolar Disease Demographics

Bipolar disease is one of the most common and severe mental illnesses an individual may be diagnosed with, but it is also one of the most confusing because there can be periods of normalcy and functionality, sometimes lasting for years, between the manias and the depressions. Bipolar is not just an American problem, in case you were wondering. The disease can be found in every country around the world and there is no race or ethnic group predilection. The World Health Organization, in assessing the global burden of this disease, found bipolar, along with three other psychiatric conditions, to be among the top 10 disabling diseases worldwide. Millions of people suffer from bipolar disease and millions more—family, friends, and coworkers—suffer with them. The overall lifetime prevalence of bipolar disease throughout the world averages between 1 and 1.5 percent. When the disease is divided into subtypes there is a lifetime prevalence rate of 1 percent for bipolar-I, 1.1 percent for bipolar-II, and a 3.0 to 8.3 percent rate for the spectrum bipolar conditions, although some researchers believe this particular statistic may be as high as 10 percent (Gartner 9). The National Institute of Mental Health (NIMH) has found that 2.6 percent of the adult population have bipolar disease and this higher percentage likely reflects increased recognition of the bipolar spectrum disorders, which may have gone undetected in earlier epidemiological studies. Men and women are equally affected, although women are more likely to have bipolar-II and rapid-cycling bipolar. The strongest predictor of developing bipolar disease is having a first degree relative—parents, siblings, or children— with the disease.

While children can and do have bipolar disease it more commonly begins after puberty between the ages of 15 and 19, although it may be mistaken for extreme teenage behavior and remain undiagnosed until adulthood. The next most common age of presentation is 20–24 and the average age of diagnosis is 21. Hornbacher describes the common pattern of a moody childhood that worsened during her teen years to finally explode in early adulthood: "The past few years have seen me in ever-increasing flights and falls of moods.... I have ridden these moods since I was a child, the clatter of the roller coaster roaring in my ears while I clung to the sides of my little car. But now, at the edge of adulthood, the madness has entered me for real" (2).

Bipolar disease can occur at any age up to around 50 and there is often as much as a 10-year delay in diagnosis, sometimes more. Although Dr. Sis had a difficult life beginning in childhood because of her undiagnosed bipolar disease and she suffered greatly from her teen years throughout her adult life, her diagnosis didn't come until she was well into middle age: "I was strange all along. You know there is something but you don't know what. So the questions 'When did it show up?' and 'When did it get diagnosed?' are about 45 years apart. Sadly." New onset of mania after the age of 50 is suspicious, suggesting causes other than bipolar disease, and a medical workup should be undertaken to discover the problem. Care must be taken to ensure that mania occurring after age 50 is indeed new onset, as some individuals may have actually had their onset as a teen or young adult, either undiagnosed or forgotten, and remained relatively stable for the majority of their adult life, only to have the disease return at this later age:

> Dawn was 54 when, out the blue, she bought a second home in another state while she was there on vacation. She then quit the job she had held for many years and moved to her new home but didn't get a new job or put her old house on the market. She proceeded to buy several cars and a boat, none of which she could afford, before her friends and family realized that something was very wrong and her actions were not just the result of a mid-life crisis. Dawn was eventually hospitalized for acute mania but not before she was ruined financially and left homeless because she had no job and no way to pay for any of her manic purchases. Although it seemed that this was a case of new onset mania after the age of 50, it was revealed during Dawn's hospitalization that she had suffered a "nervous breakdown" at age 20, and had been placed in a mental hospital for a

time. Although she was diagnosed with bipolar disease all those years ago, she had refused to accept the diagnosis and somehow managed for many years to keep her symptoms under control by self-medicating with alcohol and marijuana. Because she was highly functioning, her eccentric and passionate personality was either accepted or overlooked until she suffered her manic breakdown at age 54.

A high percentage of bipolars attempt suicide and statistics range from a 20 to 50 percent incidence of suicide attempts with a 1 to 15 percent incidence of completed suicide (Goodwin and Jamison I: 249). These rates, gleaned from studies done over the past 30 years, are felt to be double what they are today due to better available treatment, although the higher rates probably still apply early in the disease before adequate mood control is achieved. Accidental death during mania is due to risky or impulsive behavior and may appear as suicide when, in fact, suicide during mania is uncommon. The highest risk of suicide is during the mixed mood state, when depression and mania are intermingled, and the next highest risk of suicide is during the depressed mood state. The exact percentage doesn't matter as much as the fact that bipolar can be a deadly disease if left untreated, inadequately treated, or is particularly resistant to treatment.

Bipolar as a Physical Brain Disease

Each bipolar experience is unique and the path to diagnosis is too often delayed, obscured, and difficult. Any illness for which symptoms fall in the realm of emotional expression will often go unrecognized until those symptoms become so severe that the behavior driven by those extreme emotions begins to fall outside the bounds of normalcy. Even some patients with brain tumors, if those tumors affect parts of the brain involved in emotional expression, may present with altered mood states, delaying or obscuring diagnosis. Other physical illnesses may also begin with subtle symptoms that go unrecognized until they become severe enough to attract attention. How many times have we heard stories of heart attack victims who suffer for days from what was thought to be persistent heartburn? Physical symptoms, if persistent, are usually taken more seriously than emotional ones, although both types of symptoms often indicate real, biologically based disease.

We talk about heart "disease" with the gravity appropriate for a serious medical condition, but we dismiss bipolar "disorder" as if it were a problem less serious and less physical than other diseases. Untreated bipolar "disorder" can be quite deadly due to an elevated risk of suicide or the risky behaviors that accompany mania and can cause tremendous suffering and disability if undiagnosed and either left untreated or inadequately treated. The term "disorder" implies a mild mix-up in the way the body or mind is functioning while the term "disease," usually associated with specific signs and symptoms, implies a physical illness with a biological cause. I prefer the term bipolar disease over disorder because I think it best captures the true nature of this multifaceted illness. I've noticed that many sufferers either use the term manic-depression or bipolar disease when talking or writing about their illness. Clearly they, too, believe the term "disorder" fails to capture the seriousness of their illness, while others feel that manic-depression describes their illness more fully than the less emotionally descriptive word "bipolar."

There is a tremendous societal bias regarding mental illness in general and bipolar disease in particular. Most people do not understand that bipolar and its subtypes, including recurrent depressions, are almost always inherited and are therefore biologically based illnesses, although awareness of the heritability of several types of mental illness is growing. You inherited this disease from one of your parents, although they may show only subtle signs of having bipolar disease or, in some cases, no signs at all. If you look among your extended family members, you'll likely find others who fall within the bipolar spectrum even if you don't know of any who have full-blown bipolar disorder. Mark Vonnegut, son of author Kurt Vonnegut, tells of inheriting the disease from his mother's side of the family: "I can trace manic depression back several generations. We have episodes of hearing voices, delusions, hyper-religiosity, and periods of not being able to eat or sleep. These episodes are remarkably similar across generations and between individuals" (5). The genetics of bipolar disorder will be discussed in more detail in chapter 6, "Bipolar Disease Genetics," but for now, understand that you did not do this to yourself, nor did anyone or anything do this to you. You were born with the genes that predisposed you to develop bipolar disease. As Dr. Sis says, "This whole thing is absolutely not your fault. Get over that idea. This is something that has happened to you, not because of you."

Marya Hornbacher had been in and out of psychiatric hospitals since she was 16, battling anorexia and bulimia. She found herself at age 20 drunk and cutting her arms to calm her racing thoughts when, on an impulse, she cut one wrist to the bone and severed an artery. She called for help and was taken to the emergency room, sewn up, and given a blood transfusion. When asked if she needed a psychiatric hospitalization, she declined, and was then sent home. The psychiatrist accepted her explanation of the knife slipping as she was making dinner, despite the obvious fact that she had freshly carved the patterns of a leaf and snake on her arm. Hornbacher says, "They, and I, and everyone else think I'm just a disaster, a screw-up, a mess.... Surely she'll grow out of it, they think. I grew into it. It grew into me. It and I blurred at the edges, became one amorphous, seeping, crawling thing" (7). Even when faced with clear evidence of a serious and potentially deadly psychiatric problem, the psychiatrist on call in the emergency room that day completely missed the diagnosis. Because Hornbacher had been symptomatic since early childhood, her family and doctors seemed unable to separate her bipolar symptoms from her "messy" personality. They ignored the fact that her family history was full of suspiciously bipolar relatives: a manic-depressive uncle, another uncle who once painted a live horse, a great-grandfather who habitually ran off with the circus, and her own father, who had recurrent bouts of severe depression and periods of rages. Bipolar happened to Hornbacher. She was born with the right mix of genes and the right environmental triggers to activate her disease in early childhood. It was not her fault. It is not your fault, either.

When I give talks or teach a class about bipolar disease, there's always someone in the audience who experiences an "ah-ha" moment when they link up the symptoms of the disease with someone in their family, and suddenly I see anger and resentment change to understanding and compassion. To understand that bipolar disease is not just something you alone have, but that it belongs to the entire family, is to share your burden and your struggle with those who also share your DNA. If your family rejects you and doesn't want to admit the disease is an inherited, physical problem, just know that their rejection may hide the fact that they are frightened because your diagnosis hits closer to home than they want you to know. I've not seen a family yet with one bipolar member where other members of the family didn't show some form of mood disorder; you just have to know what to look for and how to ask. Had you asked me thirty years ago if my family had any bipolar members, I would have laughed at you. Today, there are definitely three, and three more from preceding generations based on family history, and who knows how many in the generations before that?

If you are searching your own family tree, look for past suicides or suspicious deaths, alcoholism or other types of substance abuse, chronic or episodic depressions, "nervous breakdowns," or evidence of psychosis, such as odd behaviors, ideas, visions, or quests. Odd or eccentric relatives in a family with other bipolar members are always suspect. Once you learn about mood disorders, you'll be able to recognize your affected family members. Your family won't get by with acting like this disease belongs to you and you alone; it's in their genetic material, too, whether they admit it or not. There are some who say that the stigma of having a mental illness is made worse by the idea that it's biologically based, that you are considered "doomed" if your biology forces you into a mental illness that you can't, by sheer force of will, overcome. While that may be true for some, I find that most people feel great relief knowing the hurtful things that are sometimes done and said during unstable times are part of a true disease causing altered thinking rather than true meanness done by people who know exactly what they are doing and saying.

Bipolar as a Chronic Disease

While you may be initially relieved to know what's wrong with you, once the reality of having a chronic disease sinks in, your relief may vanish. Managing this illness is going to require a lot of work, you may be realizing. And a part of you may be resisting the idea of having a chronic illness that will require lifelong medication and medical care. If so, you are no different from anyone who is diagnosed with a lifelong chronic physical condition. It is a difficult transition to begin to see yourself as chronically ill despite the fact that you have most likely been living with the symptoms of your illness for a long time. It is difficult to make peace with the idea that you will require daily maintenance medications—for life—in order to control your illness. But diabetics do it, heart failure sufferers do it, asthmatics do it, organ transplant patients do it, and you can do it, too.

Health can be achieved within the confines of chronic illness but only when that illness is under reasonable control. That requires close medical supervision, a proper medication schedule, and a healthy lifestyle—regardless of what that chronic illness might be. You must understand that you can never stop taking your medication, no matter how normal or good you feel. Feeling too good may even be a sign of developing hypomania and bipolars all too often stop their drugs when this happens, often with disastrous results. No matter how you feel, you must make the decision to stay on your medication, no matter what, and to discuss any medication changes you feel you may need with your doctor. One of the most difficult things about the disease is that it pushes you to want change and excitement and disruption when, to keep things under control, you need exactly the opposite. But stability and a healthy lifestyle are critical to the management of your disease. Heart patients make dietary changes and alter their physical activity, asthmatics avoid contaminated air and control their allergies, and every chronically ill patient, whatever their underlying problem, needs to live a healthy lifestyle. You are no different.

Knowledge Is Power

Now that you understand mood disorders, bipolar mood states, and the biological basis of bipolar disease itself, you have learned that there is a physical basis for your mood swings. I hope you will be able to let go of any guilt or shame you may have associated with your diagnosis. Learning that you inherited genes that made you susceptible to developing bipolar disease may not only help you accept that your illness is a physical one, but it may also help your family and friends move past blame and anger to a position of understanding and support. As you begin to assimilate this basic information, you are beginning to build the foundation for learning as much as you can about your disease. You can't just sit back and be a passive observer, knowing nothing about your disease and allowing others to manage it for you. When you are in the throes of a bad attack or recovering from a bad attack, you may have to let others have more power over your bipolar disease for a time, but your goal is to prevent those attacks from occurring so you can keep your power. And to do that you need to learn as much as you can so you will be able to manage your disease yourself.

Summary

1. Mood disorders involve recurrent, fluctuating and cyclical moods that interfere in some way with a day-to-day functioning.
2. Moods in mood disorders are often blamed on external life events when in reality the sufferer is primed to overreact to these events due to their brain dysfunction.
3. Keeping a mood chart or diary can help reveal the cyclical nature of mood swings.
4. The two main mood disorders are bipolar disease and major depression.
5. The bipolar mood states are hypomania/mania, depression, or a combination of the two, called a mixed state.
6. Bipolar disease is found worldwide with statistics ranging from 1 to 10 percent, depending on which spectrum diagnoses are included.
7. Bipolar commonly begins after puberty and is diagnosed in teens or young adults, with the average age of diagnosis at 21, but can present up to age 50.
8. There is an increased rate of suicide or accidental death in untreated or poorly treated bipolar disease.
9. Bipolar is a family disease. If you have it, others in your family have it, too, in past or current generations.
10. Bipolar is a chronic disease that requires daily medication and lifestyle maintenance to control.

Chapter 4

Bipolar Disease Diagnosis

"Manic depression is not simply flip-flopping between up and down moods.... My euphoric highs were often as frightening as the crashes from them—out-of-control episodes that put my life in jeopardy" (Behrman xxi). This is Andy Behrman's description of his bipolar, a disease that eventually crippled him yet remained relatively invisible, with symptoms elusive enough to evade diagnosis by seven psychotherapists and psychiatrists. Behrman lived the life of a successful New York art dealer by day while he roamed all-night bars and partied and abused drugs by night, performed in strip clubs, and provided young male prostitutes to his art clients. He never saw his hypomanic or manic behavior as a problem until he was arrested and put on trial for art fraud. The stress and jail time that inevitably followed brought on depression, and antidepressant treatment resulted in psychotic manias and crushing depressions that finally led to Behrman's bipolar diagnosis.

Behrman's delayed diagnosis is not all that uncommon. While his hypomanic/manic behavior—the hypersexuality, impulsivity, risk-taking, lack of judgment, and substance abuse—is typical of bipolar disease, it was overlooked again and again because of his highly functioning, party-all-night lifestyle. It's not that Behrman didn't think something was wrong. He went from therapist to psychiatrist to psychologist seeking an explanation for his out-of-control behavior, but he came in under the radar every time. Even after his diagnosis, he had to hear the word "bipolar" countless times before he was fully able to accept it.

Most people have conflicted feelings about being diagnosed, even if they know something is wrong, and Behrman was no different. They seek an answer, yet when they get what they've been looking for, they don't want to believe they have a serious mental illness. They hope for an easy fix. Perhaps a pill will solve their problem with no change in lifestyle or maybe a bit of counseling will help them work out their issues. No one wants to be told they have a lifelong condition that can be managed but not cured or that disease management will require daily medication and significant lifestyle changes. It's no surprise that many people balk at a diagnosis they didn't expect and certainly didn't want. But diagnosing bipolar disease is a complex process and is not done frivolously. It's more likely that the diagnosis will be missed, as in Behrman's case, rather than applied incorrectly. Once you get the diagnosis, don't waste your energy trying to deny you have the disease. Move past denial and accept what you have.

Diagnosis is a complex and artful undertaking based on classifying symptoms into patterns and categories. Even Kraepelin, the German psychiatrist who described and organized all the known mental illnesses in the late 1800s, recognized the difficulty in pinning down a definition that would work for each individual with bipolar disorder: "The delimitation of the individual form of the malady is in many respects wholly artificial and arbitrary" (54). This is why any attempt at categorization of bipolar disease, or any mental illness for that matter, can at times be difficult. Experience on the part of the mental health professional is a vital part of the diagnostic formula, because individuals and even their friends and family often don't recognize and therefore don't report some behaviors that are symptomatic of bipolar disease. Experienced and seasoned professionals know how to take a thorough and detailed history in order to gather as much information as possible, and they know how to observe the individual for behaviors and ways of thinking that are typical for bipolar. They know that not all cases fall neatly into the arbitrary categories listed in their diagnostic manuals. Observation of symptoms over a period of time, as well as documentation of response to medication, is sometimes needed in cases that are unclear and may take months or even years and can result in a change of the original diagnosis. In fact, this may happen more than once. Diagnosing a mental illness is more complex than diagnosing pneumonia or gout or other physical illness, simply because the symptoms of a mental illness are mostly behavioral or emotional and fluctuate over time.

As you will see in this chapter, there are tools that mental health professionals use to arrive at a diagnosis. I will focus mainly on the *DSM* diagnostic criteria because it is usually the foundation of bipolar diagnosis. The Mental Status Exam (MSE) presentation of bipolar focus on patient appearance, mood, thought content, the presence of delusions or hallucinations, suicidal thoughts, aggressiveness or violence, and judgment and insight. Each mood state will be discussed in detail, along with its *DSM* criteria and MSE presentation. Although I present an overview of bipolar categories and their symptoms in this chapter, specific information regarding your particular diagnosis can be obtained only from your mental health professional. If you are confused, have questions, or still don't understand how the criteria in this chapter apply to your situation, don't hesitate to ask your mental health professional to explain the specifics of your diagnosis to you. Only when you are confident in your diagnosis can you accept your illness and begin to manage your disease.

The *Diagnostic and Statistical Manual of Mental Disorders* (*DSM*)

The *DSM* has long been considered the "Bible" that mental health professionals use to diagnose many types of mental problems. This manual outlines diagnostic criteria and lists symptoms that are associated with each disorder in order to standardize diagnosis, but reliable diagnosis isn't necessarily accurate diagnosis. It should be obvious that mental illness categories listed in any manual represent only the current state of knowledge at the time the manual was printed. Each major *DSM* revision reflects the change in knowledge since the last revision; categories change, new symptoms or illnesses are recognized and added, and other symptoms or illnesses are dropped or defined differently. Each *DSM* begins to drift out of date as soon as it is printed. The discovery of a specific gene causing a particular mental illness, for example, could completely change the diagnostic criteria for that mental illness. Even though categorizing the complex symptomatology of mental illness is arbitrary and subject to change, doing so imposes order and continuity to the mental health field, allowing mental health professionals to communicate effectively with each other.

The History of *DSM-I* Through *DSM-IV-TR*

The first two *DSM*s, published in 1952 and 1968, didn't exactly set the psychiatric world on fire, as they were mainly a set of clinical impressions regarding various mental illnesses without any attempt at diagnostic categorization. At the time the *DSM-I* was published, bipolar disorder was called manic-depressive reaction, but when the manual was revised in 1968, the *DSM-II* renamed manic-depressive reaction as manic-depressive illness. The *DSM-III* was introduced in 1980 and its revised version, the *DSM-III-R*, was introduced in 1987. These versions contained descriptive diagnostic criteria in an effort to improve diagnostic reliability. There have been relatively minor revisions, in the *DSM-IV* (1994) and the *DSM-IV-TR* (2000), since then. From the *DSM-III* until now, changing diagnostic criteria, although minor, resulted in diagnoses that needed to be altered or refined over time. For example, one of my family members was originally given the diagnosis of schizophrenia at the time when psychosis was not thought to be a part of manic-depressive illness. This diagnosis was later changed to bipolar as the diagnostic criteria for bipolar expanded to include significant psychosis.

The Concept of Polarity in the *DSM-III* and *DSM-IV*

The *DSM-III* and *DSM-IV* versions emphasized polarity (manias and depressions) over recurrence in mood disorders, separating bipolar from major depression. This excluded highly recurrent depressions from the bipolar classification despite their original inclusion under the bipolar diagnosis. In particular, the *DSM-IV* criteria were more episode-oriented than disorder-oriented and did not take family history or past patient history into account, nor did the individual criteria carry different weights. Also, the bipolar versus unipolar classification of depression was first outlined in the *DSM-IV*, where the term "unipolar" depression described recurrent, cyclical depressions *without* manias as opposed to cyclical depressions *with* manias (bipolar). Regardless of the presence or absence of mania, those depressions were assumed to be cyclical and recurrent: if mania was present, the bipolar diagnosis was applied and if no mania was recognized, the unipolar depression diagnosis was given. Somehow, the unipolar term came to be used to describe all non-bipolar depressions, whether recurrent or not. The original description of bipolar by Kraepelin in 1899 included highly recurrent, cyclical depression even in the absence of mania, and current thinking is again moving toward classifying these types of depressions as subtypes of bipolar disease.

Although the *DSM-IV* did well to go beyond the classic bipolar definition and include a couple of subtypes of bipolar disorder, most significant, bipolar-II, excluding antidepressant-triggered hypomania or mania from the bipolar diagnosis could have potentially done the most disservice. There is little evidence to support this exclusion and there is evidence to the contrary. Every psychiatrist and mental health professional I know ignores this criteria and believes that mania induced by antidepressants is predictive of bipolar disease. My family member was originally diagnosed as bipolar-II versus severe unipolar depression and placed on an antidepressant with the warning to carefully observe for the development of mania. Six weeks later, full-blown mania and psychosis was present, changing the diagnosis to bipolar-I. For my family, and for many others, the triggering of mania from such treatment helped pin down the bipolar-I diagnosis and dispel any denial we may have had about the diagnosis.

The *DSM-V*

The *DSM-V* makes no distinction between single and recurrent episodes of major depression although it attempts to exclude single episode depressions from grief over major life events. And it once again completely separates depressive illness from the bipolar category. At least the unipolar term is gone and the antidepressant-induced disclaimer has been eliminated and a new category has been added to include bipolar mania caused by medication or depression (or mania) caused by the withdrawal of medication. Otherwise, the *DSM-V* diagnostic criteria for bipolar disease has not changed significantly from the *DSM-IV-TR*. It does not rely as heavily as previous manuals did on symptom checklists but uses dimensional assessment specifiers for disorder symptoms and severity scales, allowing for a more detailed description of the disease diagnosis. For example, a bipolar-I diagnosis might have the specifier coding of "with anxious distress" or "with rapid cycling" (71). A bipolar-II diagnosis might carry the "severe," "with mixed features," and "with mood-congruent psychotic features" specifiers (75).

Is this latest *DSM* version an improvement over the previous one? That remains to be seen. It is a working model and too new for professionals to know just yet whether it will be clinically useful. As Dr. Darrell Reiger, vice chair of the *DSM-V* task force, said, "And that's what the *DSM* is—a set of scientific hypotheses that are intended to be tested and disproved if the evidence isn't found to support them" (Brauser). If you thought the *DSM* was the "Bible" of diagnosis, that statement should convince you otherwise. This current version of the *DSM* is no more valid than any of the previous versions and it only attempts to reflect how our understanding of mental illness has changed since the *DSM-IV* was first published.

For example, the concept of spectrum disorders was unheard of in 1994; this concept may eventually prove to be false or may be confirmed and expanded as more studies are done and more data is obtained. The *DSM-V* will be revised in time and, in fact, has already received a good deal of criticism regarding its embracing of the spectrum concept of mental illness, which some believe leads to overdiagnosis. Others object to the inclusion of new mental illnesses, such as hoarding, binge eating, and hypersexual disorder (sex addiction) and Internet disorder, the latter two coming with the caveat that they require further research. Critics say that under the new or broadened categories of mental illness a large percent of the population will have a diagnosable mental illness. Regardless of this concern, the *DSM* attempts to bring order to chaos as long as it's understood that the classifications of mental illness contained within its covers are arbitrary and might well change in the future.

Mental Status Exam (MSE) and *ICD-10*

While the *DSM* is an objective and useful tool employed by mental health professionals to standardize diagnosis across the field, a sizable part of diagnosis occurs from old-fashioned observation of and talking to the person seeking a diagnosis. This is called the Mental Status Exam, or MSE. The mental health professional will observe the individual for signs of each of the bipolar mood states and note physical appearance, facial expression, and body posture and language. The individual will be asked about their inner thoughts and feelings, including suicidal thoughts and delusions. Attention will be paid to overall health as physical problems such as thyroid disease may worsen bipolar, and other medical conditions may mimic it. As each person will present with her own unique brand of symptoms, the experience of the diagnosing mental health professional is extremely important.

Other mental health professionals may prefer to use the World Health Organization's *International Statistical Classification of Diseases and Related Health Problems*, 10th revision (*ICD-10*), which lists codes of diseases and their signs, symptoms, and related information for each body system and includes a category for mental illness. The United States will begin official use of the Clinical Modification version (*ICD-10-CM*) on October 1, 2013, and all HIPAA facilities will be required to use this coding manual. The coding is included in the *DSM-V*. Whether the *ICD-10* adds to, replaces, or has no effect on the use of *DSM-V* remains to be seen.

Using the DSM and MSE to Diagnose Bipolar

The MSE is used in conjunction with the *DSM* (or the *ICD-10*) to diagnose bipolar disease by focusing on the clinical exam to determine the mental status and mood state of the person seeking diagnosis. An incomplete or inaccurate history may skew the diagnosis unless additional clinical information is available. While the *DSM* criteria serve as the structure for diagnosis, clinical observation in the form of the Mental Status Exam fills in the details. A diagnosis can be made during an initial visit, but only when an individual is able or willing to share all of their symptoms. Sometimes an initial diagnosis must be changed as new symptoms come to light:

> Roy, a 21-year-old college student who suffered lapses in memory and wild, outrageous, and embarrassing behaviors he was told about but couldn't remember, received an incomplete diagnosis because he gave an inaccurate history to his mental health professional. It was obvious to the evaluating psychiatrist that Roy was deeply depressed, but he was too embarrassed to relate the wild behaviors he

had been told about. Lacking this evidence of mania, the psychiatrist diagnosed depression, prescribed an antidepressant, and 3 weeks later Roy was fully manic, delusional, and paranoid, crouching in the corner of his dorm room, terrified of his roommate. He was hospitalized and his diagnosis was changed to bipolar-I once the complete clinical scenario became obvious.

This pattern is actually quite common. Hypomania and mania are frequently underreported, leading to initial misdiagnosis. The bipolar usually doesn't have the insight to recognize the full range of symptoms. While friends and family frequently have a better grasp of an individual's abnormal behavior, as well as any impairment that is present, especially in rising hypomania or mania, they are too often excluded from the initial assessment appointment.

Bipolar traits are intricately woven among an individual's unique personality traits. The diagnostic criteria aren't always a perfect fit. You might feel you don't completely meet the criteria for bipolar disease, but your mental health professional understands all the ways the criteria can manifest and you must trust his experience. He may simply recognize your bipolar based on gut feeling and experience. This is the "art" as opposed to the pure science of medicine. As you become better known to your mental health professional, your diagnosis might be changed, refined, or confirmed. You may not have reported all the important information your mental health professional needed to know about your situation, so a confident diagnosis could not be made initially. While there are symptoms that are shared commonly among many sufferers, these symptoms are often expressed in a unique and individual manner in each person. One size does not fit all when it comes to bipolar disease.

The *DSM* Criteria for Bipolar-I

Mania is the diagnostic mood state for the diagnosis of bipolar-I and must be present for the majority of every day for at least seven days but may be of any duration if it's severe enough to require hospitalization (65). This mood state is defined as a sustained, abnormally "up" mood that is accompanied by increased energy that leads to goal-directed activities or purposeless agitation when mania is severe. While the mood is usually "high" or even euphoric, it can be irritable, aggressive and even violent at times. Mania is usually preceded by hypomania and it may be followed by hypomania or by depression. Because major depression can exist with or without obvious mania or hypomania, it may take time to witness whether an abnormally elevated mood is associated with a depression, so a bipolar diagnosis may be delayed if no history of mania or hypomania is obtained at the time a major depression diagnosis is made. Bipolar-I mood episodes are rated as mild, moderate, or severe or with psychotic features with additional specifiers to more fully describe the mood episode. These specifiers are anxiety, rapid cycling, mixed, melancholic or psychotic features, catatonia, peripartum onset, or having a seasonal pattern (70–71). The specific criteria for the diagnosis of mania and hypomania are discussed below.

The DSM *Criteria for Hypomania and Mania*

The *DSM* diagnosis of mania requires at least three of the following criteria (four if the mood is irritable): an increase in self-esteem or grandiosity, a reduced need for sleep, excessive or uncontrollable talking, racing thoughts, distractibility, markedly increased activity (may or may not be goal-directed), and excessive pleasure-seeking despite negative consequences (65–66). Mania causes significant impairment in functioning, and if severe enough or if delusions and psychosis occur hospitalization may be required. The *DSM* criteria for hypomania are identical to those of mania, but the degree of symptomatology is less pronounced and the duration is less. Hypomanic episodes are characterized by an elevated and sometimes irritable mood lasting at least four days and symptoms generally do not cause significant impairment of functioning, although others notice a definite change in the person's usual behavior, personality, and level of functioning. For example, a hypomanic may have inflated self-esteem, while a manic has grandiosity; or a hypomanic may be able to get by on five hours of sleep each night and feel rested, while a manic may barely sleep two hours, if that much. Psychotic delusions are not present in hypomania. Neither mania nor hypomania can be due to a medical problem or substance abuse. Specific descriptions of the criteria for hypomania and mania will be discussed below. I have linked some symptoms for the purpose of discussion because they are intimately connected, such as increased activity and reduced sleep.

Inflated Self-Esteem and Grandiosity

While the hypomanic feels more confident, stronger, more attractive, smarter, and more functional than their usual self, leading them to take on challenges they normally wouldn't dream of tackling, the manic takes this to even greater heights by having delusions of grandeur. This grandiosity is characterized by an extremely exaggerated sense of self-worth that may cause the manic to feel more important than she actually is. It may result in big plans that are unrealistic or overly elaborate, such as a get-rich-quick scheme or a sudden decision to go to medical school despite the fact that the manic has never graduated from college or high school. Big projects might be taken on so that the manic becomes extremely overcommitted both at home and at work. In advanced mania, this grandiosity may combine with extreme irritability, so that the manic becomes excessively impatient and demanding or perhaps even violent in order to get what he feels he rightly deserves and has been wrongly denied. About three-fourths of manics suffer delusions, usually consistent with their inflated self-esteem. Parking spaces open up just for them, red lights turn green so they alone can keep driving, and the whole world bends over backward in order to serve them in every way possible. When something goes wrong—no parking space is available, the traffic light turns red— they erupt with anger because they see these things as a personal attack on their specialness.

Kay Jamison describes grandiosity as "feelings of ease, intensity, power, well-being, financial omnipotence, and euphoria [that] pervade one's marrow" (*An Unquiet Mind* 67). Bipolars may experience religious revelations, believe the secrets of the universe have been revealed only to them, or become convinced they have been chosen above all others to do something special to benefit all of mankind. Hornbacher describes her grandiose thinking as "not *mad* as in *moody. Mad* as in *under the impression that I am God*" (71). Keith Steadman also experienced his grandiosity in religious terms: "Delusions of grandeur manifest themselves in so many different ways. It could be Jesus Christ one day and even God on another. I tried these roles when I was flying at my highest level, both of them were great fun despite the terribly long hours and immense responsibility. The pay check never did arrive, but it was payment in itself to control the world by means of invisible buttons and psychic power" (6). Dr. Sis remembers a manic grandiose experience that occurred when she was walking home one night after lending her car to a homeless couple. She encountered an animal she had never seen before, despite having two degrees in veterinary science:

> He just walked right up to me. I said, "I don't know what the HELL you are." We just looked at each other. Then he turned and calmly walked across the road. And I said "Thanks." I perceived that I had been honored to know an animal that maybe nobody else had ever seen. My manic interpretation was that I had been "led" to this experience as a reward for helping two homeless people, and thus I was walking home at 4 a.m. and encountered my "reward." Quite a reward for an animal person to experience.

Decreased Sleep/Increased Activity

I have combined these two symptoms because they are so closely connected: as energy increases, sleep decreases or ceases altogether. Around 80 percent of hypomanics or manics have either insomnia or markedly decreased sleep. This may be an extremely productive period if the mind is hyperalert and hyperconcentrated, which is most common in the hypomanic mood state. Art is produced, books written, music scored, deals made, money exchanged, houses cleaned, grass cut, and many other activities are obsessively pursued during these energetic, hyper-focused periods. Hypomanics see themselves as productive and conscientious rather than driven. As Dr. Sis says, "We are highly functional because our brains don't know when to turn off. It's amazing what you can do if you don't ever sleep." Dr. Sis is able to intellectually perform at a high level when she is experiencing the benefits of increased energy and mental focus when hypomanic:

> I am quick and I am mentally sharp—like a razor. I do things like make a 100 percent on a doctoral dissertation. This was never done in vet. school before. I did the same thing on my Neuro. final. I made an A and everybody else but one failed it flat. I studied for 20 hours with just bathroom breaks. Energy, energy. All of my most excellent accomplishments have been inspired via this disease. I write, I compose music, I write poetry and songs, I create all kinds of paperwork and forms for my business, I create Power Points, on and on.

Many artists, poets, musicians, authors, and entrepreneurs have taken advantage of these hypomanic productive times, as you will learn more about later in the book. One notable example is Van Gogh, who suffered from cycles of mania and depression his entire adult life. He was an extremely prolific artist, producing around 900 paintings and even more drawings and sketches during his career, many of which were done during hypomanic and manic periods, particularly in the last two years of his life as his disease worsened. He attempted suicide multiple times until he finally succeeded.

This increased activity is initially goal-oriented until mania worsens to the point where purposeful activity becomes impossible as concentration wanes and distractibility increases. Productivity ceases completely when confusion or psychosis begins to dominate. Unfortunately, lack of sleep fuels the hypomania and later the mania, so the less bipolars sleep, the more manic they become and a psychotic crisis might be triggered. Every psychotic episode Dr. Sis has suffered has been due to lack of sleep when she either ran out of her prescription sleeping medication or didn't have the money to buy it. Although the hypomanic doesn't feel tired after a few nights of decreased sleep, it is vitally important to sleep in an attempt to arrest the hypomania before it rises to mania. Hornbacher describes her vulnerability to sleep deprivation this way: "The flight back was a red-eye, and that was the trigger, something that small: one night without sleep, the tiniest bit of jet lag—two hours' time difference—and I was off to the races" (259). Bipolars appear to have inherited a circadian rhythm malfunction that makes them more susceptible to sleep disruptions than other people. This will be discussed in more detail in chapter 6, "Bipolar Disease Genetics."

Excessive Talking/Pressured Speech

Excessive, uncontrolled talking, or "pressured speech," is nearly universal in manics; 80–90 percent have this symptom. What begins as rapid or nearly nonstop speech eventually becomes so one-sided and domineering that normal conversation with the manic is impossible. Cheney describes what this feels like from the manic's perspective: "There's no telling what manic lips might say, although you can be sure it will be laced with profanity and innuendo.... The urge to talk gets greater and greater ... until it's as irresistible as a sneeze in a dust storm" (67). Repressing the urge to talk is difficult and many manics find they need some type of physical action to serve as a pressure valve in order to let off steam, such as leg jiggling, finger tapping, yawning, fist clenching, or tic-like twitching. Some talk with their lips shut but with their jaws moving while never making a sound, in order to suppress their need to talk. Cheney's definition of pressured speech illustrates how forceful the urge to talk truly is: "'Pressure-cooker speech' is more like it, because unless all those unspoken words are somehow released, silence explodes into screams, and screams are not so easily ignored" (67–68). Pressured speech may take other forms. Dr. Sis describes one such episode: "One night I just started talking in rhymes. Every single sentence rhymed. I could not stop it. I could not slow down either. Hours.... They took me back to my parents' house.... I collected my medicine ... and then they took me home. An hour after I got my meds I was back to normal (not really normal, but more normal)." Sometimes this can take the form of nonstop writing, where walls, floors, furniture, or anything that a pen or pencil can make a mark on will be used to display the endless flood of words pouring out of the manic's brain.

Racing Thoughts/Flight of Ideas/Distractibility

Thought quickens, mental sharpness increases, and ideas flow with a fluidity and free association that fosters brilliance or creativity in hypomania and mild mania. Behrman explains: "My manic mind teems with rapidly changing ideas and needs; my head is cluttered with vibrant colors, wild images, bizarre thoughts, sharp details, secret codes, symbols, and foreign languages. I want to devour everything—parties, people, magazines, books, music, art, movies, and television" (xix). The hypomanic may be a sparkling dinner companion or witty conversationist, but eventually everything falls apart as mood elevates into mania. The brain begins to work so quickly that thoughts race and ideas come and go, jumping from one subject to the next with little connection to each other. The manic becomes extremely distractible, which interferes with the ability to process and actually use the ideas and "epiphanies" that are produced during mania. Cheney describes flight of ideas, or racing thoughts, this way: "Manic epiphanies are like shooting stars: flashes of brilliance that are gone in an instant" (101). Concentration can't be trained on anything for very long; ideas, even brilliant ones, are gone almost as quickly as they come and the mind is on to the next idea, and the next, and the next. No one can think as fast as the hypomanic can until the speed gets out of control in mania, as Kay Jamison described it: "The fast ideas are too fast, and there are far too many; overwhelming confusion replaces clarity.... Everything previously moving with the grain is now against—you are irritable, angry, frightened, uncontrollable" (67). Mania at this point may deteriorate into psychosis, a mixed episode, or a depressive state.

Excessive Pleasure-Seeking

Increased pleasure-seeking behavior is common and can take many forms, from risky sexual behavior to gambling to drug and alcohol abuse to extravagant spending to fast driving. Behrman describes his pleasure-seeking behaviors in terms of living life with passion, "taking second and sometimes third helpings on food, alcohol, drugs, sex, and money, trying to live a whole life in one day" (xix). Impulsive buying that maxes out credit cards and drains bank accounts will predictably plunge the manic deeply into debt. Jamison says, "When I am high I couldn't worry about money if I tried. So I don't. The money will come from somewhere; I am entitled; God will provide" (*An Unquiet Mind* 74). Drug and alcohol abuse may occur not just for self-medication purposes but purely for pleasure-seeking, and impulsivity and risk-taking add to the mix, leading to dangerous, destructive behavior, as Behrman describes: "The symptoms of manic depression come in different strengths and sizes. Most days I need to be as manic as possible to come as close as I can to destruction, to get a real good high—a $25,000 shopping spree, a four-day drug binge, or a trip around the world. Other days a simple high from a shoplifting excursion at Duane Reade for a toothbrush or bottle of Tylenol is enough" (xix).

Risky, dangerous behavior while manic may seem like suicidal behavior but technically isn't intended as self-harm. It may either be a way to feed the mania or a desperate attempt to dampen the manic high, which Cheney describes after she slashed her wrist to the bone and severed an artery: "I didn't necessarily want to be dead, just dormant for a while.... Manic feelings are sometimes so brutally strong is seems like there is no way to endure them" (97).

More than half of manics are hypersexual, with an inflated sense of their own sexual attractiveness, as Cheney describes so well: "If there was one sure sign of mania's approach, it was this secret conviction I got that I was the ultimate arbiter of other people's sexuality, this sudden rush of confidence that no man—or woman, if I so desired—was beyond my jurisdiction" (40). Manics or rising hypomanics may undertake an atypical sexual encounter—a heterosexual may engage in a homosexual liaison, for example—or seek out multiple partners, have unprotected sex, or initiate an affair if married. They may cross all sorts of boundaries and initiate inappropriate sexual contact with children, teens, congregation members, patients, students, neighbors, or friends' spouses. This does not mean that these individuals are pedophiles or sexual predators when they are not hypomanic or manic. In the throes of hypersexuality, judgment and insight disappear and anyone is fair game. Once mania wanes, hypersexuality also wanes and the desire for inappropriate sexual contact evaporates, as Allan's case demonstrates:

> Allan was a 44 year old car dealership mechanic who had spells of feeling "up" with increased sexuality that disappeared when his mood waned. During these periods of elevated mood, he would often begin an affair and leave his wife and teenage daughter to move in with the object of his current passion. Once his mood returned to normal, he ended the affair, moved back home, and resumed his normal family life. He worked extra hard to provide for his family and to make up for the time he had been away, eventually taking to his bed from "exhaustion." Allen was unaware of a family history of bipolar until the suicide death of his daughter, when his mother confessed that she had been diagnosed with bipolar years before but had kept this a secret from the family. She had been suspicious about his spells of exhaustion, which she suspected might be periods of depression, and had been watching him closely for signs of mania but hadn't seen his multiple affairs as a sign of bipolar disease, thinking instead that "men will be men."

Impulsivity/Lack of Judgment/Risky Behavior

These symptoms overlap with many of the previously mentioned symptoms. Impulsivity is so common in mania that it is considered one its prime features and, in fact, appears to be present in bipolars even when they aren't manic, suggesting this characteristic may represent a fundamental trait of the disease in addition to being a symptom of the manic mood state. Impulsive behaviors may present in many ways, such as taking extreme physical chances like driving recklessly, attempting daring and crazy stunts like trying to beat a train over the railroad tracks, or jumping off roofs or out of windows. Bingeing on drugs or alcohol, excessive shopping, impulsive travel, and cutting and other self destructive behaviors may occur on a whim. It's not surprising that accidental deaths sometime occur due to these risky behaviors, but these deaths are not to be confused with suicide. When an idea pops into the head of a manic, they act on it without a second thought. They may buy a new car, move to a new town or state, hop on a plane with no idea where they are going or what they are going to do when they get there, quit their job, get married to someone they barely know, or break off a relationship, all on a whim. They may disappear without warning, leaving distraught family and friends behind to worry about their fate, as Katie's story illustrates:

> Katie was a 26 year old retail clerk who had several previous hospitalizations for suicidal depression during her teens and early twenties. She had done well for a few years and was working and living on her own when her parents got a call from her employer asking why she hadn't come to work all week. Katie's worried parents quickly drove to her apartment and found her in a catatonically depressed state; when she refused hospitalization they took her home where they could care for her. Within a week she had disappeared and they had no idea where she was until 2 weeks later when they got a call from an emergency room halfway across the country, informing them that their daughter was acutely manic, had been stopped by the state highway patrol going over 100 mph, and was being involuntarily committed. Her diagnosis was changed from chronic depression to bipolar-I.

Judgment is generally good in mild hypomania, although it tends to be a bit expansive, leading hypomanics to take on more projects and commitments than they normally would, which they can usually handle until their hypomania worsens and they begin to inch closer to mania while their judgment begins to slip. By the time they have reached mania, they have seriously impaired judgment leading to disastrous consequences financially, at work, and in their personal relationships. This lack of judgment in manics can be shocking, invariably involves risky behavior, and is nearly always associated with grandiosity, pleasure-seeking, and sometimes delusional or psychotic thinking. Retirement or savings accounts may be invested in risky get-rich-quick schemes, snap decisions to move or change jobs may impulsively be acted upon, and professional or social overcommitment may occur with disastrous consequences. As Cheney points out, any sense of boundary or appropriate behavior is lost once mania takes hold: "There's a fine line between almost manic and mostly manic, when charmingly indiscreet turns into just plain indiscreet, and seductive becomes obnoxious.... [T]hat line always gets fainter and fuzzier the closer I get to mania, until eventually there is no line, there never was a line, and any line that might have been disappears altogether, along with all of my discretion and judgment" (67).

Behrman began to sell counterfeit artwork despite the fact that he was a legitimate dealer for the successful New York artist he was counterfeiting, made hefty commissions from the sale of this artist's work, and was a trusted insider in the art business. In a stunning lack of insight and judgment, he dealt with his regular clientele when selling his fakes, so he left a trail of paperwork that was easily traceable to him. As his mania increased, his judgment declined to the point where he viewed his actions as merely an elaborate and ironic joke on the artist rather than a criminal act. He was ultimately convicted of conspiracy to defraud.

The MSE Description of Hypomania and Mania

The MSE description of mania and hypomania reflect differing degrees of elevated mood or irritability as observed by the mental health professional. The hypomanic is nearly always "up," while the manic is inappropriately elated or euphoric. Their clothing, jewelry, makeup, or hairstyle may be too bright, too sexual, too odd, or too attention-seeking. They may look as if they have thrown everything on in a hurry, as if they can't be bothered to slow down enough to close all the buttons or zippers. The hypomanic person appears energetic, optimistic, productive, confident, and full of plans, while the manic individual takes this to the extreme by having an overinflated opinion of himself or his abilities. He sees himself as having an extremely active mind or as being extremely creative or social. The rising hypomanic and manic appear hyperactive, restless, disorganized and flighty. They may talk, walk, and do everything fast. Although their thought processes are quite rapid they are extremely distractible and can't stay on one idea for long. While hypomanics can be irritable, impatient, pushy, and aggressive at times, manics can be extremely irritable, impatient, and even violent if provoked.

Hypomania

As mood begins to rise from a depressed or normal mood state, a person usually becomes hypomanic before they enter the manic mood state. Particularly after emerging from a bout of depression, entering a state of hypomania may be perceived as simply feeling good after a prolonged period of feeling bad. Such a "recovery" from a depressed mood state is not likely to be viewed for what it really is—yet another mood state. Hypomania can be difficult to recognize simply because hypomanics possess qualities that our society admires and rewards. Who would ever think that a confident, happy, optimistic, energetic person, full of plans and ideas, who manages a great number of responsibilities, may be showing signs of a mental illness? If spells of hypomania alternate with periods of depression, this pathologic mood state becomes more apparent, but persistent hypomania or hypomania alternating with small dips in mood can be very difficult to detect. There is evidence that some individuals may have prolonged periods of hypomania without any dips in mood, representing a subtype of bipolar called functional hypomania.

Terri Cheney recognized when the hairs on her arms and neck would "ripple with pleasure like wind-stroked wheat" (32) that hypomania was beginning: "Oh my God ... the little hairs ... they were my manic trip wires. Inevitably, when the chemical balance in my brain started to shift, they were the first to alert me to it.... I knew that it was hypomania, heavenly hypomania at last" (32). Most bipolars describe the hypomanic state as their best, happiest, and healthiest self, and struggle with the less creative, energetic and productive self that emerges when they are not hypomanic, often refusing to believe that their hypomanic persona is merely a mood state and not who they really are. Cheney says that when hypomanic "the world was suddenly all about textures and tastes and sensations, too many and too much to be ignored. It was all so wickedly delicious, actually the best part of being bipolar" (32).

Bipolars crave their hypomanias, when energy levels are high, sleep requirements drop to only three or fours hours a night, and they wake each morning feeling refreshed and enthusiastic about whatever the day may bring. Life lived this way is full of wonder and promise; the temptation to reduce or terminate medication in order to induce or prolong this heightened mood state is strong. Certainly the will to increase medication to terminate this mood state is nonexistent. The hypomanic loses insight as their self-esteem rises and their judgment becomes impaired and they begin to edge closer and closer to mania, as Cheney describes: "I was perfect ... because I was perfectly hypomanic: three-quarters of the way to mania, at that point where all things ... seem utterly fascinating. I don't need candlelight ... because I am naturally incandescent. If I smiled at you, you caught the glow. If I touched you, you felt the fire" (141). It's hard to keep a perspective of the entire scope of the disease when this mood state is so pleasurable, but what goes up continues to go up, and then must inevitably come down.

Mania

Mania is characterized by a euphoric, elevated mood with increased cognition and sensory perception that Dr. Sis describes like this:

> You can see and hear and sing and do absolutely everything on a completely different plane. Lights, sound, every ticking clock, every dripping faucet, the hum of fluorescent lights.... All your senses are on fire, or firing. You see things with new clarity. You hear things that everybody tunes out. Higher and lower frequencies. Higher and lower wavelengths of light. Intense colors! Intense music! Miracles are everywhere. There is emotional intensity, too. Great epiphanies. Religious experiences. Life magnified a thousand fold.

Behrman describes mania in similar terms: "Manic depression for me is like having the most perfect prescription eyeglasses with which to see the world. Everything is precisely outlined. Colors are cartoonlike, and, for that matter, people are cartoon characters. Sounds are crystal clear, and life appears in front of you on an oversized movie screen" (xxi). Behrman says mania is like being in Oz, with all its color and excitement, while being sane is like finding yourself back in Kansas, with its monocolor landscape and boring, everyday existence. He says that when he's manic, even the sound of his eyelashes beating against his pillow is like thunder. Keith Steadman describes being manic like this:

> Being high on the back of mania is the best feeling there is, the best fun, the best of everything and a whole lot more besides. It is a place where every sensation and emotion are tirelessly breeding new sensations and emotions, whose sole purpose in life is to work devotedly at raising the beholder up to a paradise tantalizingly close to where mankind is really intended to be, an existence that perhaps we may all have been sharing as normality today if Adam hadn't managed to go and cock things up for us all by munching on that blessed big apple [4–5].

Michael Greenburg's daughter, Sally, suffered an acute manic attack with delusional psychosis at age 15. She was hospitalized with a bipolar-I diagnosis and received intensive outpatient psychiatric care upon discharge because her mania was difficult to control. This is what Greenburg remembers Sally's psychiatrist telling them about mania and then specifically describing mania in terms that Sally could relate to:

> [M]ania is a glutton for attention. It craves thrills, action, it wants to keep thriving, it will do anything to live on. Did you ever have a friend who's so exciting you want to be around her, but she leads you into disaster and in the end you wish you never met? You know the sort of person I mean: the girl who wants to go faster, who always wants more. The girl who always serves herself first and screw the rest.... I'm just giving you an example of what mania is: a greedy, charismatic person who pretends to be your friend. We may not be able to resist her every time, but one of the things we're going to try to learn is to recognize her for what she is [172].

Just as Sally's psychiatrist warned, mania, and hypomania are seductive and difficult to resist and they may be difficult to recognize in the early stages, but they are easily recognizable in their most severe, delusional, or psychotic manifestation. Dr. Sis says, "It is hard for me to tell that I am going manic. I can pretty well see it when I am in full mania, but I have trouble seeing it coming [because] it comes in on little cat feet." Physical activity increases and may transition from energetic and purposeful activity to hyperactive, driven behavior and finally to bizarre, inappropriate, or psychotic acts. When the bipolar is enjoying feeling good, has plenty of energy, and is performing well at home and at work, it's understandable why denial may set in about becoming hypomanic. Many, if not most, bipolars do not think their hypomanic states are a big problem and may not see any reason to intervene until things worsen. Even

Dr. Sis feels this way: "It is very important to me that I can voluntarily bring myself to the edge whenever I need to perform, but not fall off. My performance when hypomanic is so excellent and so inspired that I am willing to risk going over the edge."

Hypomania may be so prolonged and so productive and relatively normal in appearance that the slide to mania may catch everyone by surprise, as Marilyn's story illustrates:

> Marilyn was a 35-year-old homemaker with three small children who had suffered significant postpartum depression after the births of each of her children. After the birth of her third child, she had seemed more energetic and happier than usual once her depression lifted. Marilyn's husband had recently become concerned over the hours she spent on the computer after the children were in bed for the night. He knew about chat rooms and suspected she might have gotten involved in an Internet romance. Marilyn eventually spent so much time at her computer that she began to stay up all night. When her husband tried to talk to her about it, she argued that she kept the house clean, the children cared for, and meals on the table so she was doing her job and he needed to leave her alone. One night, Marilyn's husband slipped into the computer room unnoticed and discovered that she was looking at pornography on the Internet, which surprised and confused him, but he decided not to make an issue of it since his fears of an on-line romance weren't true. As she stayed up night after night, Marilyn became increasingly irritable, restless, and obsessive about the house staying clean. One day as he was coming home from work, Marilyn's husband found her walking in the snow along the road to their house, naked. The children had been left unattended, unfed, diapers unchanged, crying for hours, but safely locked in their rooms and left in their baby beds. Marilyn was hospitalized and diagnosed with acute, psychotic mania and bipolar-I disorder with a postpartum onset.

Marilyn had a common postpartum bipolar onset, which unfortunately took three pregnancies to be recognized. Her goal-oriented hypomanic activity was geared to caring for her children and her home, while her pleasure-seeking and hypersexuality took the form of Internet pornography. When she became acutely manic and psychotic, however, she was no longer able to maintain her household chores and childcare. Fortunately, she made sure her children were safe in their rooms, even as they were left neglected for the day.

The manic might feel a sense of connection with the world or nature, or with mankind and all creation. This may take the form of mystical or religious experiences. Physical sensations of pain, cold, and heat may be blunted while sensations of pleasure are heightened; the manic can be outside in the very cold weather without clothes, like Marilyn in the snow, or walk on rocks without shoes or move through brambles without discomfort. The sense of well-being one feels when hypomanic reaches a crescendo in mania, yet irritability inevitably creeps in. Hostility towards family and friends might be expressed if they try to intervene on the manic's behalf. Even when flying high, an underlying restlessness and mood instability is present and ready to erupt with little provocation. The manic has an inflated sense of importance and has difficultly understanding why people aren't treating them with the respect they feel they deserve—why can't others see how important they are? Sexual excitement may be intense and lead to affairs or other sexual gratification outlets, such as Marilyn's Internet pornography obsession.

Nearly all bipolar memoirs concentrate on mania and manic escapades and this makes for interesting reading. It is amazing how far mania can escalate before such behavior attracts enough attention to require intervention, either by law enforcement, family, or other authority figures. Manic individuals may be seen as promiscuous, high-stakes party people, hyperactive wheeler-dealers, and extremely sociable individuals, but these behaviors are overlooked as long as the person is able to function on some level, no matter how poorly, in their daily life. Certainly their lifestyle and the culture and community in which they live play a role in how much leeway they are given in their behavior. A person living in New York, for instance, may be able to live a wildly sexual life that is easily kept hidden from most of the people he associates with during the day, as Behrman was able to do. A person living in a small town who carries on a series of affairs cannot expect her behavior to be kept secret. A person living an artistic lifestyle, such as an actor, writer, artist, or musician, would likely be given more behavioral freedom than a preacher, teacher, or doctor.

Mania can be quite complicated at times. It differs from person to person and each person can have a different pattern of symptoms during each manic attack, although symptoms generally follow the same pattern. Nearly half of manics are also depressed (called a mixed mood episode), two thirds are euphoric, and almost three fourths are irritable (also mixed). Mood is extremely changeable during mania, with only a small percentage of people— 5 percent—showing any sort of stability of mood. Women, in particular, are more likely to have quick dips into depression.

In the past, mania could cause stupor, a kind of catatonic state of the brain if not the body. This was a rare and very serious form of mania called delirious mania (or Bell's mania) where severe delusions, hallucinations, paranoia, and disorientation suddenly occurred. These people did not sleep or eat and became extremely debilitated and died from exhaustion after months of hyperactivity. When you read about deaths from mania or manic exhaustion in historical or literary texts, Bell's mania is most likely the cause. This form of mania is thought to be where the expression "raving maniac" came from. Because available treatment of bipolar disease over the years has left fewer people untreated, there has been less interest in this category of mania, which is now considered to be archaic. However, one researcher concluded that this condition may still exist today, although it is less pronounced and is more likely from chronic psychosis than from mania alone.

The DSM *Criteria for Depression*

For a diagnosis of depression, the *DSM* requires a major depressive episode to last at least two contiguous weeks and include at least five symptoms, one of which must either be a depressed mood or a loss of pleasure or interest in activities that the individual previously was interested or engaged in. Diagnosis requires at least four additional symptoms from the following list: a significant change in appetite or weight, with either increased or decreased appetite and a corresponding weight gain or weight loss; a change in the normal sleep pattern, with either increased or decreased sleep; a change in activity level, with either agitated activity or retarded movement; fatigue or loss of energy; tortured thoughts of worthlessness or guilt; concentration difficulties or indecisiveness; or persistent thoughts of death or suicide including suicidal plans or a suicide attempt. These symptoms must cause significant difficulty in daily functioning as well as emotional distress and cannot be the result of substance abuse or a medical condition (67–78).

Bipolar depression represents the opposite mood state as compared to mania, with feelings of worthlessness as opposed to those of well-being or grandiosity and a general slowing down rather than a speeding up of thinking, speech, and energy. There is little if any interest in sex as opposed to the hypersexuality of mania, with a lack of the ability to experience pleasure as opposed to the heightened pleasure-seeking behaviors of mania. Psychosis with delusions and sometimes hallucinations can occur in severe depression but are less common than in mania. Delusions usually match the depressed mood state and consist of financial, physical, or spiritual ruin; for example, the person may feel that he has sinned and deserves to be punished. Paranoid delusions, with feelings of persecution, may occur but are more likely to be seen in mania.

There are many symptoms of depression and each person will have her own unique expression of the *DSM* criteria. For example, the change in sleep pattern may take several forms. There may be difficulty falling asleep, or a person may wake up in the middle of the night or very early in the morning, or sleep excessively yet constantly feel tired (a common pattern in bipolar depression). While the actual variation of the sleep pattern might be different for each person, the fact that a sleep pattern change will occur is extremely likely. There may be variation in a person's normal diurnal rhythm so that a depressed person may wake up feeling worse in the morning, feel progressively better during the day, and feel best in the evening. A loss of sexual drive is very common.

Depression nearly always takes the more somatic form of physical tiredness or aches and pains, either real or imagined, without a sense of sadness or despondency, although feelings of melancholy may occur and accompany this pervasive lack of energy. An existing physical condition may seem to worsen or new symptoms may pop up, many or which are hypochondriacal in nature. If psychosis occurs, there may be the sensation of rotting internally or the belief that one has an undiagnosed fatal illness. For example, the British Romantic poet William Wordsworth, who was violent and moody by his own description, and was most likely bipolar, suffered from various maladies that had no physical basis. His biographers confirm that he suffered from severe depression.

MSE Description of Depression

The MSE description of depression reflects both the physical appearance and activity level that signal this mood state and the thought processes that result from it. The depressed person will often appear to have taken very little time or trouble getting bathed or dressed. Both men and women may wear wrinkled, sloppy, or poorly fitted clothing if they have gained or lost weight due to changes in appetite. Their hair may be unstyled, uncombed, or unwashed and they may not have bathed in days. Men may have unshaven faces and dirty hands and fingernails and women may wear no makeup or jewelry. Depressed people may move and talk slowly (psychomotor retardation) in a quiet, monotone voice, appearing tearful and sad, or they may seem anxious, worried, and jumpy. Their faces appear sad or vacant and they may have poor to no eye contact as they express feelings of hopelessness, helplessness, and feeling dead inside. Their thoughts are overwhelmingly negative and often focus on death or other morbid topics, including suicide.

Depression

Guilt seems to be ever-present in depression; and even when it's not delusional, it can be overwhelming, causing the bipolar to obsess over all the ways he is lacking in life. This rumination accompanies a general slowing down of all the cognitive brain functions so that the depressed person feels foggy and stupid, with poor memory and concentration. Irrational fears begin to take over and obsession with sin and religious matters may occur, regardless of the bipolar's previous religious beliefs. People with depression may become extremely judgmental about themselves and their lives, convinced they have either broken religious rules or are unable to follow them properly. Life loses all meaning and nothing they do matters anymore, if it ever did. They believe they are utterly and completely worthless. Steadman describes the unrelenting, day-in and day-out torture of depression like this:

> Maddening, sickening repetitive hogwash flooded my nights, until it was officially time to rise and step into another daily horror story.... Depression certainly isn't pretty. It is capable of sending the most violent and disturbing thoughts through one's head. I used to feel like a prize fighter who had taken a terrible beating. My already out of joint nose gets sent first class to a different part of my face, and my mind is blown to pieces, yet there I was, still taking punches left right and centre, never allowed out of the ring except in a body bag [258].

As depression deepens, there is mental and physical slowing so the person is unable to accomplish normal, everyday activities, as Cheney describes: "My body simply refused to obey my mind's commands. I just lay there—unwashed, uncombed, and drowning in inertia, struggling with the need to breathe in and out" (178). Depression may deepen to the point of utter hopelessness, to where no joy can be found in any part of life, and the bipolar sincerely believes that even those closest to them would be better off if they were dead. A significant number of bipolar suicides occur during the depressed mood state. Steadman described his suicidal thoughts like this:

> *Never* laugh at the absurdity or size of a depressed person's overblown problems.... Why does depression refuse to clock out? Grey thoughts tramped through my body, bleeding pain into snarled bed sheets throughout the night. My mind's destructive buttons was always pushed well in, my knobs were fully turned, and my levers were pulled all the way down, providing me with the rotten sensation of being subjected to a terminal five minute warning every two sickening seconds. I tried praying to God to let me go, to be my latest killer, to close the lids of my eyes and also the lid of the cardboard coffin, glued together with sticky stigma, wrapped in brown paper, tied up in black ribbon and topped off with a sweet maraschino cherry [257–58].

When I first read J.K. Rowling's *Harry Potter and the Prisoner of Azkaban*, I believed the evil Dementors added a chilling new psychological layer to this fantasy series. The description of the Dementors left me in no doubt they were meant to embody suicidal depression. I have since learned that Rowling has suffered severe depression in the past and created those monsters as a result of her experience. She describes the Dementors as draining all positive emotion and memory out of people, leaving only despair and horrible memory in place of the good. The victim is said to be left empty, with no hope of recovery, without thought or a soul, in an existence described as worse than death. The physical sensations that Harry feels when a Dementor is near are chilling; actual contact with a Dementor is horrifying. Harry seems to be particularly vulnerable because of his troubled childhood, which included being orphaned after witnessing the murder of his parents. Other characters in the book suffer the typical "lows" and stresses of life and are thus more resilient, making Harry a prime target for the Dementors.

Judgment is impaired and insight is often lacking in depression, although not as much as in mania; planning is difficult and depressed individuals may forget to pay their bills, including their mortgage or car payment. They may stop going to school or work because they have difficulty concentrating and they may see no point in tackling routine, everyday tasks because they have no hope for the future. They may feel detached, doomed, singled out for punishment, and powerless to defend themselves. The mind obsesses with tormenting thoughts of personal failure and worthlessness, suicidal thinking is extremely common, and the risk of suicide is quite high. Homicide followed by suicide may occur, particularly when the suicidal person perceives the world as hopeless for themselves and those closest to them. Depression may be obvious to others, but some individuals are able to hide their depression remarkably well until their suicide eventually exposes their hidden torment, as Mary's unexpected suicide demonstrates:

> Mary, the 17-year-old daughter of Allan the mechanic, was a troubled high school student. School officials believed her father's many absences as well as his bed-ridden "exhaustions" when home contributed to Mary's rebellion against male authority while her poor school performance was due to ADD. Although she was moodier than the typical teenage girl, she could be gregarious and loving among her friends. Mary's father came home after work one day to find her unconscious and fatally hemorrhaging with multiple cut marks on her arms and slit wrists. Everyone was shocked by Mary's suicide—no one had suspected anything was wrong as she had not seemed depressed and had appeared excited to attend a school dance that weekend. Mary's grandmother had suspected her grand-daughter and son might be bipolar but she wasn't sure, as neither seemed to exhibit the highs and lows that she herself had suffered throughout her life. She had been afraid to speak out because she didn't want anyone to know about her own diagnosis.

Bipolar memoirs do an excellent job of describing the hypomanic and manic states, but depression is too often given few pages and little description until it reaches suicidal levels, at which point the suicide attempt is described in detail. Perhaps it is felt that readers need help in recognizing and understanding the hypomanic and manic mood states since they are so frequently misunderstood or overlooked. Often there's nothing much of interest to write about during a depressed mood state as compared to manic antics. Perhaps writers don't want to revisit their depressions in order to write about them. One of the best descriptions of depression was written by Pulitzer Prize-winning author William Styron, who described his suicidal depression in chilling detail:

> The gray drizzle of horror induced by depression takes on the quality of physical pain. But it is not an immediately identifiable pain, like that of a broken limb. It may be more accurate to say that despair, owing to some evil trick played upon

the sick brain by the inhabiting psyche, comes to resemble the diabolical discomfort of being imprisoned in a fiercely over-heated room. And no breeze stirs this caldron, because there is no escape from this smothering confinement, it is entirely natural that the victim begins to think ceaselessly of oblivion [50].

This was Styron's first experience with depression but he would have another severe episode 15 years later that came after a period of mood swings. His second severe depression manifested in physical complaints that changed on a daily basis and confused his doctors so that he was placed in an ICU for a time before the psychological nature of his psychosomatic complaints was eventually discovered.

Nearly everyone understands depression on some level but bipolar depression can be quite different from the situational depressions that are experienced by non-bipolars, so accurate descriptions are important. Jamison says: "Depression is awful beyond words or sounds or images; I would not go through an extended one again. It bleeds relationships through suspicion, lack of confidence and self-respect, the inability to enjoy life, to walk or talk or think normally, the exhaustion, the night terrors, the day terrors" (*An Unquiet Mind* 217). Those without mood disorders usually get depressed for a specific reason—a lost job or loved one, the diagnosis of a serious illness, a financial setback, or a romantic breakup. They feel sad, lonely, frightened, or lost and they need time to regroup as they adjust to their loss. Most people are able to grieve, adjust, and move on with their lives in time. Bipolars are often crushed beyond all description and can't even begin to rally for recovery. That is why suicide often seems the only way out.

Bipolar depression may come without warning and reason, as Cheney describes: "Like most of my chemical depressions, this one came out of the blue, like a freak electrical storm in the middle of a sunny summer afternoon" (178). Because bipolars' depressions are biological and not normally a reaction to life, sadness is not always experienced, as Behrman points out: "Contrary to what most psychiatrists believe, the depression in manic depression is not the same as what unipolar depressives report. My experience with manic depression allowed me very few moments of typical depression, the blues or melancholy. My depressions were tornadolike—fast-paced episodes that brought me into dark rages of terror" (xxi). Milder bipolar depressions may appear as pervasive dissatisfaction aimed at oneself or one's life or anything associated with it, such as job, spouse, social status, or financial situation.

Mixed Episodes

A mixed episode results when the depressed and manic mood states occur simultaneously. For example, an agitated depression may be called a depression with mixed features (agitation) if depression is predominantly present. Even in mania, there may be moments of depression, when a switch to a depressed mood state is near. At other times the mood mix seems about equal. Because of this variability of symptoms, the most accurate definition of a mixed state reflects the rapid switches between euphoric mania and severe depression, which Cheney describes so well: "From the moment I awoke, and every minute thereafter, I had been a quivering mass of volatility: up, down, irate, flirtatious, contentious, giddy, seductive, paranoid" (75). Hornbacher also describes the rapid switching of a mixed mood state: "Rage swings until a stuporous sleep, and sleep swings into the awful morning sun ... my mood plummets from shrieking high to muffled low" (57).

Once considered rare, the mixed state is now recognized as being quite common. Features vary, depending on severity; psychosis may or may not be present, judgment and insight is severely impaired, physical aggression may be displayed, and suicide risk is high. Delusions and hallucinations occur more frequently in the mixed state than in the depressed state. Women seem more prone to mixed states than men. Men or women with substance abuse, particularly alcohol abuse, seem to have a higher incidence of mixed states than those without that history. Current thinking suggests that agitated depressions should be considered mixed depressions, consistent with the idea that recurrent depressions represent a subtype of bipolar disorder.

Bipolars describe this state as being so intolerable suicide often seems the only way out and, in fact, three-fourths of all bipolar suicides occur during mixed episodes. Hornbacher describes mixed states as "episodes where both the despair of depression and the insane agitation and impulsivity of mania are present at the same time, resulting in a state of rabid, uncontrollable energy coupled with racing, horrible thoughts—people are sometimes led to kill themselves just to still the thoughts" (6). Jamison describes her switch from mania to depression with mixed features like this: "I can't think, I can't calm this murderous cauldron, my grand ideas of an hour ago seem absurd and pathetic, my life is in ruins ... my body ... raging and weeping and full of destruction and wild energy gone amok.... I understand why Jekyll killed himself before Hyde had taken over completely" (*An Unquiet Mind* 114).

The *DSM* Criteria for Bipolar-II

The *DSM* criteria for bipolar-II require that one hypomanic episode must be met along with a major depressive episode, either current or in the past (see specific criteria for hypomania and depression as listed under bipolar-I diagnosis). Symptoms must be clinically significant, with disruption of normal functioning, and not the result of a medical condition or substance abuse. There cannot have been a previous manic episode, as that will give a diagnosis of bipolar-I. The same severity and descriptive specifiers used in bipolar-I are used in bipolar-II (74–75). Individuals who have suffered highly recurrent depressions may find themselves in this diagnostic category and may respond better to bipolar medication than antidepressants. The hypomanias may be difficult to recognize after emerging from a period of depression but careful history-taking should reveal their presence. This diagnosis is discussed in more detail in chapter 5, "The Bipolar Spectrum."

The *DSM* Criteria for Cyclothymic Disorder

Diagnosis requires subthreshold hypomanic and depressive symptoms, meaning these mood stages do not completely meet the *DSM* criteria for hypomania or major depression, over at least a two-year period. These mood states must have been present at least half the time and cannot have not been absent for more than two months at a time. There can be no medical causes or substance abuse causing these mood episodes and some degree of functional impairment or personal distress must be present (76). When you begin to evaluate subthreshold symptoms, there can be difficulty in differentiating normal from abnormal behavior, so this can sometimes be a difficult call on the part of the mental health professional. If an individual has a family history of bipolar and has symptoms of excessive moodiness or substance abuse, has moved from job to job or town to town, has had multiple affairs or marriages, or has a quick temper or a mercurial temperament, this is good evidence that this individual might be cyclothymic.

This diagnosis falls within the spectrum concept of bipolar disease, which some mental health professionals reject, believing that widening the net for diagnosis of bipolar disease sets the bar for diagnosis too low. But cyclothymics suffer for their excessively moody personalities and they often heap a great deal of suffering on those connected with them. While their functioning may not be as impaired as bipolar-I or bipolar-II individuals, their erratic and unpredictable personality causes its own type of impairment.

The *DSM* Criteria for Specified Bipolar Disorder

This category is used when a bipolar diagnosis does not completely meet the standard bipolar-I or bipolar-II categories. It embraces the bipolar spectrum concept and allows the mental health professional some leeway in diagnosis, particularly early in the diagnostic process when the full picture or a complete history of the illness may not yet be known. Individuals with this diagnosis may be changed to a more specific diagnosis over time. Clinical scenarios include hypomanic episodes of short duration (three or fewer days) along with at least one major depressive episode, episodes that don't fully meet the other criteria for hypomania or mania (other than duration) with at least one major depression, hypomania without depression or mania, and cyclothymia of less than two years' duration (81–82).

The *DSM* Criteria for Unspecified Bipolar Disorder

This category was previously called "bipolar NOS" and includes those cases that don't meet the criteria for either bipolar-I or bipolar-II but in which symptoms are still more characteristic of bipolar than they are any other diagnosis. The mental health professional may choose to use this diagnosis until further information is known about the patient, as in an ER setting, or when he may choose not to specify the reasons the bipolar criteria are not met. This can serve as a "holding pattern" diagnosis and will be changed as more information about the patient's disease becomes known (83).

Summary

1. Each *DSM* reflected the current state of knowledge of mental illness at the time of publication.
2. Categorizing mental illness is arbitrary and artificial but it allows standardization, order, continuity, and effective communication between mental health professionals.
3. The Mental Status Exam (MSE) is based on clinical observation and taking a thorough and complete history from the person seeking a diagnosis.
4. Mania must be present for 7 days and hypomania for 4 days in order to diagnose bipolar-I.
5. Grandiosity, decreased sleep, increased activity, excessive talking, racing thoughts, distractibility, pleasure seeking behavior, impulsivity, lack of judgment, and risky behavior are symptoms of mania.
6. Hypomania and mania differ only in degree and duration.
7. Depression has to be present for at least two weeks and exhibit either a depressed mood or a loss of pleasure or interest in activities that have been previously enjoyed.
8. Other symptoms of depression are a change in appetite or weight, a change

in sleep, a change in activity level, a loss of energy, difficulty concentrating, and suicidal thinking.

9. Mixed mood states include elements of both mania and depression.
10. Bipolar-II, cyclothymic disorder, specified and unspecified bipolar disorder are alternative categories of bipolar disease.

Chapter 5

The Bipolar Spectrum

For many years it was believed that only 1 percent of the population had bipolar disease and you will still see that statistic in books today. But it is becoming more and more apparent that from 30 to 70 percent of recurrent depressions belong on the bipolar spectrum, just as Kraepelin originally suggested (Akiskal). The relatively recent discovery of bipolar-II as an explanation for recurrent depression expanded that original statistic from 1 percent to 5 percent. If you add an additional 6 percent incidence for cyclothymic temperament (Chiaroni, Hantouche, and Gouvernet), which has been studied and validated as being part of the bipolar spectrum, and also include hyperthymic personality types, you will end up with a statistic that suggests one out of every 10 people will fall somewhere on the bipolar spectrum (Akiskal, Bourgeois, and Angst). This seems to be a reasonable and possibly conservative estimate. This does not mean that everyone on the spectrum has symptoms that disrupt their lives, although many do. Some of these symptoms are positive and enhance the lives of those lucky enough to be on the mild end of the spectrum.

The more open the criteria for diagnosis, the less reliable a diagnosis will be, and certainly every moody person doesn't deserve a bipolar spectrum diagnosis. The challenge, then, is to come up with a way to differentiate cyclical mood disturbances from normal variations of moody personalities. The concept of the bipolar spectrum originally encompassed a range between classic bipolar-I on one end of the continuum and recurrent depression on the other. Currently the continuum encompasses bipolar and depression as well as their variants, including traits that define certain temperaments associated with mood disorders. There is no question there are clinically significant bipolar spectrum disorders and the closer a variation is to the classic manic-depression/ bipolar-I definition, the more likely it is to be recognized and therefore diagnosed. Some variations are mild and could be classified as subclinical or subthreshold disorders, while others fall somewhere in the middle and show cyclical variations but don't fit the classic up and down mood swings we associate with bipolar disease.

The *DSM-IV* and the *DSM-V*, as well as the *ICD-10*, included diagnostic criteria for a couple of the spectrum disorders that are diagnostically distinct, but the full scope of the bipolar spectrum is not completely represented in the *DSM-IV* or the *DSM-V*. The problem facing researchers today is how to pin down clinically significant spectrum disorders that fall somewhere between the classic, severe, yet relatively uncommon bipolar-I on one end of the spectrum and the relatively common cyclothymic or subclinical/subthreshold hyperthymic personality type on the other end. How best to classify these subcategories is debatable and a consensus definition of the bipolar spectrum is still being discussed at this time. More research needs to be done before a definitive classification and diagnostic criteria can be agreed upon. I will give you the current state of knowledge concerning the bipolar spectrum in this chapter with the understanding that this area of research is evolving rapidly.

The Concept of a Disease Spectrum

A disease spectrum is defined as a group of disorders that falls under a particular disease category with a range in symptom severity. Although asthma isn't considered a true spectrum disorder I'd like to use it as an example of a disease with a common underlying pathophysiology but with different clinical presentations. When we think of asthma, wheezing immediately comes to mind and the bronchospasm that causes this wheezing is certainly one of the prominent features of this condition. While contraction of smooth muscle narrows the small airways to cause wheezing, the cells that line the interior of the airways swell and begin to produce mucous, further narrowing the airways and contributing to the wheezing. This is called an inflammatory reaction and it is one of the underlying components of an asthma attack, along with airway muscle spasm. It is also responsible for the symptoms of shortness of breath, coughing, and delayed pneumonia from abundant mucous in the small airways and air sacs of the lungs. Even when the bronchospasm has been successfully treated, this inflammatory reaction continues and is subclinically present when the patient has no obvious symptoms.

There are variable factors that trigger an asthma attack and symptoms vary from attack to attack and from person to person. Some people are wheezers with less inflammation than bronchospasm while others have a predominantly inflammatory reaction, produce a great deal of mucous, and present with an asthmatic bronchitis form of the asthma "spectrum" because they have more inflammation than they do bronchospasm. Some have only a nighttime cough while others cough during, and for a month or so after, every upper respiratory infection (this has been called cough asthma). While all of these presentations are considered asthma, they vary widely in severity and course and some presentations even have their own special terminology, but they all share the same underlying pathophysiology (airway constriction and inflammation), just in differing degrees of severity. Therefore, a spectrum of clinical presentations exists for this one disease.

In psychiatry, a spectrum disorder is more broadly defined as a group of conditions that are linked in some way; for example, a common set of clinical symptoms may be present or there may be a common underlying cause. Clinical severity may vary from severe to mild and may include subclinical or even nonclinical manifestations along the continuum. For example, the autism spectrum consists of autism on the severe end, and Asperger's syndrome on the mild end, with highly functioning autism closer to the Asperger end of the spectrum (the *DSM-V* has eliminated these specific, descriptive terms). In between those specific categories are all grades of severity; there are mild, moderate, and severe Asperger individuals as well as mild, moderate and severely autistic individuals. In addition, Asperger traits can be seen in those who don't fully meet the Asperger criteria, suggesting a subthreshold manifestation of Asperger syndrome, with these individuals at the near-normal end of the spectrum. In much the same way in the bipolar spectrum, there will be hyperthymic people with no mood disorder disability on the near-normal end of the spectrum and full-blown bipolar-I individuals on the opposite, severe end, with a great deal of variation in disease presentation between those two extremes.

The Bipolar Spectrum Disorders

Kraepelin intuitively understood the concept of spectrum disorders as he observed, organized, and then systemized his data on mood disorder patients. This is why he included all mood disorders under the umbrella of manic-depression. He observed the constant flux of mood states, from mania to depression and all the possible combinations of moods found in mixed states. Many of his patients with depression, if followed long enough, would eventually develop periods of hypomania, and some depressed patients had family histories of manic-depression or manic psychosis. Kraepelin became convinced that the underlying cause of mood disorders was a constitutional (inherited) mood dysregulation that could lead to any number of possible clinical outcomes. Thus the idea of the bipolar spectrum was born. Mania, depression, psychosis, mixed, changeable and even normal moods—it could all be there on the spectrum for those who inherit what we today call mood dysregulation, or a cycloid temperament. There is genetic support for these bipolar disorder manifestations that give the bipolar spectrum its range and variability. Twin studies of bipolar patients confirm this range from manic psychosis to the moodiness of the cycloid temperament.

The *DSM-IV* and now the *DSM-V* do not fully reflect the idea of the bipolar spectrum, nor do they make any connection between a predisposing mood dysregulation temperament and any form of bipolar disorder. If you find yourself not quite fitting the *DSM* criteria, or aspects of your condition break the "rules" of classic bipolar-I disorder, you may recognize yourself in the following descriptions of the bipolar spectrum disorders. If so, you are not alone. The *DSM* misses many a bipolar that doesn't meet its exact criteria. Cyclothymic individuals, for example, might be diagnosed as histrionic or borderline, with the emphasis on a flawed character rather than a true mood disorder. This seems particularly unfortunate in light of the fact that their underlying mood disorder is treatable. Just because these individuals aren't high enough on the spectrum scale to rate a diagnose of one of the known, classic bipolar diseases doesn't mean they don't suffer significant social and interpersonal difficulties because of their mood dysregulation. There is predictive value in identifying these "soft bipolar" disorders, particularly in juveniles, a third of whom go on to develop full-blown bipolar-I or bipolar-II disorder from their baseline cycloid temperament (Akiskal, Rosenthal, and Rosenthal). Perhaps early intervention in the form of treatment or avoidance of hypomania-inducing antidepressants could ultimately decrease the percentage of future progression to full-blown bipolar disease. At the very least, close observation so the change from cyclothymia to bipolar, should it occur, will be detected early would serve to minimize the negative consequences of untreated disease.

Classification of the bipolar subtypes is best done by first classifying underlying inherited temperament as either the cycloid (cyclothymic) temperament or the hyperthymic type, depending on expressed emotion, reactivity, impulse control, circadian rhythm, and energy level. Both the hyperthymic type and the cycloid temperament appear to represent lifelong personality dispositions. While hyperthymia rarely develops into any form of bipolar disease, cyclothymia often precedes bipolar-II (Perugi, Akiskal and Micheli). Not all cyclothymics develop bipolar disease, however.

The cycloid temperament, present in 0.4–6.3 percent of the population, can present as either predominantly depressive, hypomanic, or up-and-down/mixed cyclothymic mood states that are not so severe as to warrant a bipolar-I or bipolar-II diagnosis but are strongly correlated with behavioral and emotional problems (Goodwin and Jamison I:85). These individuals are often described as overly sensitive or moody, irritable, aggressive or even explosive, nervous, agitated or high-strung, and there is often comorbid alcohol or drug abuse. There may be episodic, cyclical behaviors exhibited, such as sexual affairs, gambling or spending, shifting sleep patterns or daytime productivity variations, and changing interests or plans or sociableness.

The hyperthymic type is stable, adaptive, and psychologically resilient, full of energy, optimistic, with an enthusiastic outlook on life, and lacking cycles of depressed mood or hypomania. These individuals tend to be warm, extroverted and social, cheerful and confident, and full of plans and ideas (Jamison, *Exuberance* 130). They are also articulate and talkative, uninhibited, and are stimulus seekers but not risk takers. Hyperthymic versus hypomanic symptoms are one of degree; feeling "up" as compared to feeling exuberant, being optimistic versus overly optimistic, and being articulate as opposed to overly talkative represents the range between these two categories. Also, being confident versus bragging and overly confident, being energetic versus overly energetic and needing little sleep, being full of ideas and plans rather than being overcommitted with activities, being extroverted or over-involved versus meddlesome, and feeling carefree and uninhibited as compared to taking risks are other ways in which hyperthymia and hypomania differ. Hyperthymic traits may remain within the range of normal behavior, but those individuals who edge too close to hypomania are at high risk for developing bipolar.

After classic bipolar-I, the remaining spectrum disorders are linked by hypomanic variations superimposed upon the cycloid (cyclothymic) temperament or (rarely) the hyperthymic type. There are four basic types of bipolar spectrum disorders as well as intermediary types that fall between these bipolar subcategories. Bipolar-I is classic manic-depressive illness; bipolar-II is recurrent depression with spontaneous mild hypomanias; bipolar-III is recurrent depression and hypomania as the result of antidepressant therapy; and bipolar-IV is depression in a hyperthymic temperament or in functioning hypomania. The intermediary bipolar types are bipolar_ or schizobipolar disorder, bipolar-I_ with recurrent depression along with a few bouts of prolonged hypomania, bipolar-II_ with depression in a cyclothymic temperament, and bipolar-III_ with recurrent depression during substance abuse (Akiskal). The possibilities for bipolar spectrum disorders do not end here; other cyclical problem behaviors may eventually be included somewhere along the spectrum.

Bipolar-I, Bipolar-I_, and Bipolar_

When we talk about bipolar as a spectrum disorder we consider the classic bipolar-I diagnosis as its most severe manifestation although there is considerable variation in its severity or any of its other features. Bipolar-I demonstrates the classic manic and depressive cycling mood states with psychosis sometimes occurring during mania and rarely during depression. Men, in particular, seem to be predominately manic rather than depressed and often have the underlying hypomanic form of the cycloid temperament. Women, who are usually more depressed than manic, often have the underlying depressed cycloid temperament and will usually continue that trend when they develop bipolar-I. Their manic mood states will usually be dysphoric or mixed. Bipolar-I_ patients appear to be most closely linked to bipolar-I. They have frequent depressions with a few prolonged hypomanias (lasting weeks), do not get psychotic, or have significant social dysfunction. Bipolar_ is a rare form of the bipolar spectrum that represents a cross between schizophrenia and bipolar-I disorder.

Bipolar-II and Bipolar-II_

Bipolar-II features depressive episodes without full-blown manias or mixed states. Hypomanic episodes occur but may be so mild as to be nearly unrecognizable and are often mistaken for feeling better after a period of depression. Episodes can occur rapidly (rapid cycling); a patient can go to sleep depressed and wake up hypomanic, convinced that a good night's sleep was responsible for the overnight change in mood. It's no surprise that some of these patients are diagnosed with major depression rather than bipolar since the depressive mood state dominates the barely recognizable hypomanic state. These depressions can be quite severe, and since rapid cycling is so common, there are many more mood episodes in this form of bipolar than might be seen in the more classic bipolar-I manifestation. Bipolar-II_ is even more unstable, with cycles of depression and irritable hypomanias piled on top of an already dysregulated cyclothymic temperament. This form of the bipolar spectrum disease is therefore more severe than bipolar-II and the unstable mood state in these patients causes a great deal of trouble for them and their family and friends. There may be associated panic disorder and social phobias and these extremely dysregulated individuals can be suicidal. These are the patients who often end up with a borderline personality diagnosis rather than a bipolar diagnosis.

Bipolar-II was the first spectrum disorder to be included in the *DSM*; however, the diagnostic criteria was overly restrictive and missed many cases of this disorder. It appears the most common form of this subtype of bipolar presents with hypomanias that are less than the 4 days required by the *DSM* to make the diagnosis. More cases would be diagnosed if a 2 day hypomania criteria was used instead. In addition, a frequent presentation of bipolar-II demonstrates cyclothymic type depressions, which commonly exhibit panic and social phobia symptoms as well as suicidal thinking, rather than full blown depressions. There is some evidence that panic attacks in the context of bipolar-II disorder may represent a distinct subtype of bipolar spectrum disorder.

Bipolar-III and Bipolar-III_

Antidepressant-induced hypomania, or bipolar-III, belongs on the spectrum despite the fact that its existence had been excluded by both the *DSM-IV* and the *ICD-10*. This exclusion has been dropped from the *DSM-V* bipolar criteria. Other treatments that induce hypomania fall into this category as well, including ECT (shock treatment), light box therapy, and sleep deprivation. Many of these patients have an underlying dysthymic or depressive temperament and have a family history of bipolarity. Fortunately, these induced hypomanic states are brief and aren't likely to recur spontaneously. The bipolar-III_ patient's recurrent depressions will always be difficult to differentiate from their underlying substance abuse and it requires a careful history to establish years of mood swings within the context of a bipolar family history to know if an underlying mood disorder exists beneath the substance abuse or is present because of it. If no family history is uncovered or if there is no evidence of a cyclothymic temperament or mood disorder prior to the substance abuse and recurrent depressions, then bipolar-III_ may be more confidently diagnosed.

Bipolar-IV

Depressions that occur in an individual with hyperthymia or with persistent hypomania with little or no dips in mood (functional hypomania) comprise this category of the bipolar spectrum, particularly if there is a family history of bipolar disease. Typically the depression associated with bipolar-IV is of late onset (past age 50), comes after years of functioning hypomania, and quickly transitions into a mixed state of agitated depression. These individuals are often successful male entrepreneurs who have benefited from their stable hyperthymic or hypomanic state, which differentiates them from bipolar-II individuals who only have brief, discrete episodes of hypomanias. This baseline hypomanic state results in the individual's possessing extraordinary drive and ambition, confidence, and boundless energy and enthusiasm. They often possess remarkable interpersonal skills, driving their achievements and successes to great levels. It is only when depression intrudes upon the hypomanic state that a mixed state results, and these successful, achieving, functioning hypomanics do not tolerate any loss of functioning or any decrease in their normally elevated mood state. This form of bipolar is particularly dangerous from a clinical standpoint. The successful stockbroker jumping to his death from his office window might be attributed to this form of bipolar. The *DSM* has no category for this expression of bipolar disease and individuals with functioning hypomania might be diagnosed as having narcissistic personality disorder.

Possible Bipolar Spectrum Behaviors

There are cyclical mood alterations that may eventually be included in the bipolar spectrum category. Seasonal recurrent depressions (without hypomanias), periodic irritability, a cyclical variant of bulimia, episodic obsessive-compulsive symptoms, or an out-of-the-blue suicide crisis not associated with an ongoing depressive state may indicate spectrum disorders. Any behavior that appears to have periodic exacerbations, including gambling, sexual addiction or other impulse control problems, is also suspect. Episodic sleep complaints, recurrent, brief depressions (not related to the menstrual cycle) and cyclical nervous complaints may also fall into the bipolar spectrum category. In addition, agitated depression, postpartum depression (particularly with psychotic features), antidepressant-resistant depression, and other types of atypical depressions including those with physical or hypochondriacal complaints, or any depression in an individual with a bipolar family history are likely to be part of the bipolar spectrum. These variants of depression often respond poorly to antidepressant therapy and respond better to mood stabilizers. Further study will be needed to confirm how many of these conditions will eventually qualify for inclusion in the bipolar spectrum.

The Bipolar Spectrum: Entrepreneurs, Immigrants, and the Protestant Prophets

When you read about prominent bipolars in this book, you will discover some amazing accomplishments the individuals who are bipolar or are on the bipolar spectrum have achieved. You will learn that family members of those with bipolar disease are often blessed with creativity, energy, drive and optimism and they, too, often accomplish great things in life. It was once thought that a gene for creativity was linked to the gene for bipolar disease and it was a lucky family member that got the creativity but not the bipolarity. We now know this is not quite the way it works. We understand bipolar disorder results from the actions of multiple genes that produce a range of symptoms from mild to severe so those family members with creativity and drive and energy are most likely exhibiting a mild or subclinical manifestation of the bipolar spectrum because the creativity trait is part of bipolar itself. The positive traits that stem from hyperthymia or persistent mild hypomania in these subclinical bipolar family members may be extremely attractive to others, as these individuals often have a great deal of interpersonal skill and charm as well as ability. Hyperthymic traits in particular tend to be quite adaptive and contribute to psychological resiliency during tough times. Yet the children of these subthreshold bipolars may be bipolar-I or bipolar-II, as the genes may be more fully expressed in future generations.

John D. Gartner, author of *The Hypomanic Edge,* interviewed a group of Internet company CEOs and showed them a list of hypomanic traits the CEOs considered not only accurate but highly descriptive of themselves (Gartner 1–6). Gartner suggests that American entrepreneurs are, on the whole, hypomanic. These highly achieving men suddenly understood their driven natures, their wild ambitions, and their boundless energy when explained in terms of hypomania. While these traits contributed to the individual successes of these CEOs, they are part of a larger picture. Our identity as a nation is tied up in such optimism, zeal, and the quest to follow our dreams, no matter how unlikely we are to succeed.

Gartner believes we are a hypomanic nation because we are formed from a population of immigrants who needed drive, optimism and risk taking to be able to leave their old lives behind in order to start a new life in a new country. There is evidence of a higher than normal rate of bipolar disorder among immigrants; countries with the highest percentage of immigrants have the highest incidence of mania. America, New Zealand, and Canada have the highest rates of mania and also the highest percentage of immigrant-based population. Asian countries, who have very few immigrants, have the lowest mania rates, while Europe appears somewhere in the middle, both in the number of immigrants and in the number of manics in the population (Gartner 11–12).

The religious conversion experience, where depression or despair allows a person deep insight and revelation, and is followed by life-changing euphoria or ecstasy, can be described as a mood-swing religious event. This was first described in *The Varieties of Religious Experience,* written by William James, who did not feel this psychological explanation of the conversion experience diminished its importance or validity (174). In fact, he felt suffering was vital to the transformative experience if one was to seek out the ultimate truths of life and death. James, a bipolar himself, studied many famous religious men and women and found this mood-swing religious pattern in all of them. The "Protestant prophets" (Gartner 35) of early America—Puritans John Winthrop and Roger Williams and Quakers George Fox and William Penn—guided their followers by force of their religious hypomanias and messianic beliefs to build a new civilization that would attract fanatics and rebels of all sorts for generations to come. Gartner suggests the religiously extremist Protestant population of early America had a high incidence of the bipolar spectrum because that type of individual may have sought the strict rules of their religion and the firm guidance of their leaders to keep them in line.

John Winthrop organized the Great Migration from England to form a "New Israel" in New England. The Puritans made sure to invest either their lives (those that went to New England) or their money (those who stayed in England) in this new venture and, in time, land was eventually owned or money was made, so their entrepreneurial spirit was as strong as their religious spirit. The hypomanic and grandiose Winthrop told his people they could defeat thousands, that their mission was to redeem the world, and that they would become a beacon of light, leading the world's people to God. But they landed in New England in the middle of winter and 200 soon died, including Winthrop's own son, who drowned the day they landed. Yet Winthrop's mood never wavered and his city on the hill, Boston, thrived over the next decade.

When Roger Williams arrived in Boston, Winthrop was thrilled to have such a saintly man join his mission, so he gave him the highest pastoral position in the city. But Williams soon found fault with both the church and with Boston itself; neither church nor city was godly enough, in his opinion. A man of sometimes ridiculous as well as volatile opinions, Williams's hypomanic mind was likened to a "windmill whirling so fast that it set itself on fire" (Gartner 43). Williams moved to a church in Salem and, after Winthrop intervened there, moved to Plymouth and then back again to Salem, where he held the position of teacher rather than pastor. At this point his grandiosity led him to personally attack the king of England in a letter, calling him a blasphemer and a liar, claiming he lacked the power to give land grants in America. The Massachusetts court stood ready to take action when Williams, on the advice of preacher John Cotton, backed down.

Williams was eventually made pastor in Salem and gave his church an ultimatum: either they separate from all the other churches in Massachusetts or he would separate from them. The Salem church did not back Williams and he was brought to court and sentenced to banishment from Massachusetts, which he was able to delay for a few months because of the harsh winter and an illness he was suffering at the time. Williams saw himself as being persecuted like Christ and he violated the conditions of banishment by preaching in his home, which he had been forbidden to do. The court decided to arrest Williams and deport him to England, where he stood a good chance of imprisonment or death, but he escaped before he could be arrested. Surprisingly, Winthrop rescued Williams and afterward they became lifelong friends and neighbors.

In an abrupt about-face, Williams, who had previously preached extreme separatism, founded Rhode Island, or "Rogue Island" (Gartner 48) on the principle of religious tolerance. Any religion (or lack of religion) was accepted. Individuals were expected to obey civil laws but otherwise experienced true freedom of religion and beliefs, or what Williams called "soul liberty" (Gartner 49). When the Quakers arrived in America, they were beaten, starved, tortured, and even hanged; the lucky ones were not allowed to get off their boats once they arrived in America and were sent back to Europe. But Williams allowed the Quakers into Rhode Island, despite pleas from the other colonies for him to refuse them entry, and so they arrived in great numbers.

Williams eventually became irritated that the Quakers had taken over most of the political offices in Rhode Island because they made up the majority of the population, so he felt compelled to challenge George Fox, the British founder of the Quakers, to a religious debate when Fox visited Providence, Rhode Island. Fox was already headed back to England when he heard about the challenge, or so he claims. It seems likely that Fox had no intention of debating Williams, knowing it would be a one-sided and unfair display of power, or perhaps he wasn't emotionally capable of going against a hypomanic when he, himself, was a predominately depressed, volatile, and elderly individual. Fox had suffered from mood swings since the age of 19, with periods of deep depression alternating with religious ecstasy. He would sometimes do bizarre things on impulse, claiming a direct mandate from God. The elderly Williams was undeterred by the absence of Fox, however, and arranged for a debate with the local Friends instead. His endless, hypomanic four-day debate exhausted the Quakers, who eventually gave up arguing their side and begged for an end to the debacle.

William Penn became a Quaker in England during a period of depression and was thrown out of Oxford for openly criticizing the school as sinful. After a long vacation in France, courtesy of his father, he returned to England uninterested in religion but years later converted again and this time it stuck. He traveled with Fox and evangelized, was imprisoned four times, and had his inheritance taken away from him. When it was against the law for the Quakers to worship in their meeting houses, Penn began to preach in the street and was arrested for disturbing the peace, but his impassioned plea swayed the jury and he was found innocent. The king of England owed a large debt to Penn's late father, so he settled the debt by giving Penn a large tract of land in America, hoping, of course, that he would rid England of those pesky Quakers in the bargain. He asked that the land be named after Penn's father but Penn had hoped to call the land Sylvania. So a compromise was struck and the land would be called Pennsylvania. Penn took Williams's idea of religious tolerance to a new level of complete religious freedom. Philadelphia was built to Penn's hypomanic ideals with an urban design ahead of its time. The Quakers proved to be worthy entrepreneurs and they soon became successful. Despite the fact that Penn owned more land than anyone, he did not enjoy financial success and landed in debtor's prison. Tenants refused to pay their rents to Penn and his financial and political authority was continually challenged in his tolerant and independent settlement. Still, Quaker Pennsylvania, and Philadelphia in particular, thrived and ultimately became more successful than Boston and New Amsterdam (New York).

Summary

1. Including spectrum disorders raises the population bipolar rate to 10 percent.
2. Widening the bipolar diagnosis criteria makes diagnosis less reliable.
3. The *DSM* doesn't include the full range of spectrum disorders.
4. Kraepelin intuitively understood the concept of spectrum disorders when he included depressions in the manic-depression category.
5. Classification of bipolar subtypes begins by noting the underlying hyperthymic or cyclothymic temperament.
6. Cyclothymics often develop bipolar-II, while hyperthymics usually remain happily resilient and adaptive throughout their lives.
7. There are four main types of bipolar spectrum diagnoses and their intermediary categories: bipolar_, bipolar-I and bipolar-I_, bipolar-II and bipolar-II_, bipolar-III and bipolar-III_, and bipolar-IV.
8. Bipolar-III encompasses hypomania induced by antidepressants or other treatments while bipolar-IV is a late-onset diagnosis in longstanding hypomania, when a mixed state of agitated depression occurs.
9. Problem behaviors that have cyclical exacerbations may one day be included in the bipolar spectrum category.
10. Various subtypes of depression, including treatment-resistant and agitated depression, are most likely bipolar spectrum conditions.

Chapter 6

Bipolar Disease Genetics

There is no question that bipolar disease clusters in families and twin, adoption, and family studies strongly suggest that bipolar disease is an inherited condition in up to 93 percent of cases. First degree relatives (parents, siblings, and offspring) of bipolars have up to ten times the chance of developing bipolar disease as compared to the rest of the population; and if one identical twin has the disease, there's an increased chance that the other twin will develop the disease at some point during their lifetime with heritability around 80 percent (Shih, Belmonte, and Zandi). There's also a genetic association between bipolar disease and major recurrent depression, supporting its inclusion in the bipolar spectrum. First degree relatives of a bipolar have three times the chance of developing depression as compared to the population at large and if one individual in a set of identical twins has bipolar disease, the other twin has a an increased chance of developing recurrent depression as well as bipolar disease. Despite these tantalizing clues of a genetic cause for bipolar disease, no study has precisely pinned down how bipolar disease is inherited and no definitive "bipolar gene" has been found.

Many studies have been done in many different ways over the years in an attempt to unravel the mystery of bipolar disease heritability. Sometimes it appears as if the disease is more likely to be passed down from the mother's side of the family, sometimes from the father's. Many different genes have been studied and many implicated. Some have been linked to schizophrenia, psychosis, panic attacks, anxiety, hyperactivity, attention deficit disorder, age of onset, and lithium responsiveness. When all is said and done, it appears that heritability of bipolar disease is extremely complex and involves at least three, and likely many more, separate genes, all of which carry their own "susceptibility factor," which taken together, add up to cause the disease.

If many susceptibility genes are involved in the inheritance of bipolar, each family likely has their own special combination of genes, which may explain why the disease is different in some families than in others (for example, why some families have clusters of suicides while others don't) or why the marriage of two bipolars or a bipolar and a chronic depressive may produce a different or worse disease manifestation in their offspring than the family has previously seen. These genes may also get duplicated as they are passed on to the next generation, amplifying disease manifestation so that the disease expression worsens in a family over generations. A person may likewise inherit the genes yet never manifest the disease because those genes were never fully expressed; most were never activated due to lack of environmental triggers or epigenetic influences (alterations in how genes are expressed without changing the genes themselves).

Basic Genetics

It should be clear that the inheritance of bipolar isn't as simple as the Mendelian genetics we learned in high school biology class, where eye or hair color, for example, could be explained by dominant and recessive alleles, meaning different or alternative forms of a gene. This is a very simple inheritance pattern where a single trait is passed down to a child by a pair of alleles that come from the parents, one allele from each parent. The inherited trait is determined by the interaction of this allele pair. There is a dominant and a recessive allele for each trait and it takes a recessive allele from each parent for the recessive trait to be expressed. When a dominant and recessive allele are paired, or when two dominant alleles are paired, the dominant trait will always be expressed. For example, both my parents had black hair, which is the dominant hair color trait, but they carried the recessive blond hair-color allele, which produced a blond child in one of their three children—me.

But even this example of Mendelian genetics is not quite that simple. What about brown hair, the color of my sibling's hair, or those children who are born with blond hair but whose hair turns brown as they reach their teens? What about the various shades of blond? Are there other alleles involved or are epigenetic factors at work here? If you have a disease that relies on multiple alleles of a gene to be expressed, then things get complicated, but if a disease requires multiple genes in order to be expressed, then things becomes very complex indeed. Some diseases are inherited via one gene and one gene only, like sickle-cell anemia and Huntington's chorea, but bipolar disease has not proven to be in that category. When my relative was diagnosed some years ago, it was believed at the time that there was one bipolar gene responsible for the disease but that other genes stabilized or destabilized that one gene, contributing to whether it was expressed or not. Researchers were hard at work back then looking for that one, definitive gene. Instead of finding "the bipolar gene," they uncovered hundreds of suspect genes that they have been studying ever since.

The theory today isn't all that different from the one gene theory; it just has a different emphasis and involves more genes, each exerting a small influence over disease expression. Instead of one major gene that is expressed or not expressed, it appears that many genes directly contribute to the final expression of bipolar disease. Think of being dealt a poker hand—just the right combination of cards in your hand will determine if you win or lose the round. In much the same way, the genes you are dealt (from your parents) may determine whether you get bipolar disease or not, and then how it will manifest in you. Were you dealt a royal flush (bipolar-I) or just a high card (hyperthymic personality)? Perhaps you got a full house instead (bipolar-II). The more genes there are, the more possible hands you could be dealt. Future research will, it's hoped, determine if a handful of genes are more important than the rest in the inheritance of bipolar, with the others contributing in some way to disease expression, or if some of the genes are linked so they are inherited together.

But inheriting these genes isn't the full story: they must be turned on before they begin to do their work. These susceptibility genes appear to require certain environmental or other triggers to be turned on. Switching these genes on appears to be relatively easy in some individuals and rather difficult in others, depending on which genes (and how many copies) a person may have inherited. An individual can inherit the genes for bipolar yet never get the disease because those genes were never switched on. Yet they can pass those genes to their children, who may fully manifest some form of bipolar disease. I've seen some people who clearly inherited the genes, with a bipolar family history and a bipolar child, who had every environment trigger possible, yet their bipolar was never activated. What protects these people and not others? It is hoped ongoing genetic research will answer this question, among others, in time.

Family Studies

Before scientific genetic studies were done, one had only to look at family trees to see that bipolar disease and its variations congregated in families. For example, the poet Alfred, Lord Tennyson, was born to a family riddled with mental illness. His father was classically bipolar and became insane at the end of his life. Of Alfred's 10 living siblings, only one was psychologically normal. The rest either had recurrent depression, cyclothymia, or strange personalities with either religious or spiritualism obsessions. One brother was classically bipolar and died from exhaustion during mania. Alfred suffered from severe recurrent depressions, although he may have had mild hypomanic episodes and today he would be most likely be classified as bipolar-II. His bipolar father's siblings were either depressed or hypomanic and their father, Alfred's grandfather, suffered from unstable moods and had a volatile and unpredictable temper (Jamison, *Touched with Fire* 198–99).

The German composer Robert Schumann developed mood swings by the time he was 18. His father, August, had a nervous breakdown the year Schumann was born and never fully recovered. His mother had recurrent depressions, his sister and a paternal cousin committed suicide, one of Schumann's sons became a morphine addict, and another went mad in his early twenties and spent the remainder of his life in an asylum (Jamison, *Touched with Fire* 206). This is an example of parents with mood disorders combining their genetics to produce worsening disease in their offspring and beyond.

Virginia Woolf had an equally interesting family history, with a cyclothymic father and a depressed mother. One paternal aunt had recurrent hypomania and a paternal cousin was bipolar and died of mania. Of Virginia's three siblings, two had recurrent depression and one was cyclothymic. Virginia was classically bipolar and committed suicide at the age of 59 by stuffing the pocket of her overcoat with a large stone and walking into the river near her home, where she drowned (Jamison, *Touched with Fire* 227). Again, this is an example of combined parental mood disorder genetics, with all of the children from this union suffering from a mood disorder. Only Virginia had classic bipolar-I, which was passed down from her father's side of the family, but her mother's mood disorder genes surely contributed to the mix.

Early genetic family studies did not separate bipolar subtypes or differentiate highly recurrent, early onset depression from less recurrent forms of depression. Data from current studies sheds more light on the genetic basis of the various subtypes of bipolar disease. A large study done in 1982 revealed that if a family has one bipolar member, the other members of that family have a 4.5 percent lifetime risk of developing bipolar disease, as compared to no risk in the control group (families with no bipolar members). The risk of developing bipolar-II disease in families with a bipolar-I member was 4.1 percent as compared to a risk of 0.5 percent in the control group. The risk of depression was 14 percent as compared to 5.8 percent in the control group and, finally, the lifetime risk of having any sort of mood disorder in the family of a bipolar-I was 23.7 percent, as compared to 6.8 percent in the control group. As a general rule, if one parent has any type of mood disorder, the children have a 27 percent lifetime risk of also having some form of mood disorder. Having both parents with a mood disorder equates to a 74 percent lifetime risk (Gershon, Hamovit, and Guroff). The genetic pattern of mood disorders and bipolar is therefore quite obvious.

Twin and Adoption Studies

While studies of family trees and psychological examinations of current family members may uncover information about the genetic clustering of mood disorders in families, environmental and socioeconomic factors as well as common family experiences or traumas can and do contribute to the triggering of bipolar disease. Since twins share the same environment but only identical twins share the same genes, their study, particularly when one develops bipolar disease and the other doesn't, helps to more fully explain the contribution of genetics in mood disorders. Comparison with non-identical twins, who share the same environment but not the same genes (and are no more related than any other siblings) further enhances the differentiation between genetics and other factors regarding the expression of bipolar disease.

Early twin studies showed that when testing for manic-depression, identical twins had a concordance rate of 77 percent as compared to a rate of 23 percent in nonidentical twins. Heritability (a product of comparing the concordance rates of both sets of twins) was 0.71, with a value of 1.00 implying complete heritability and a value of 0 implying no heritability. Later studies showed a 63 percent concordance rate in identical twins as compared to a 13 percent rate in nonidentical twins, with 0.78 percent heritability (Goodwin and Jamison II: 419–20). A study that separated out the various bipolar types found an 80 percent concordance rate in identical twins having bipolar-I as compared to 13 percent in nonidentical twins, and a 78 percent concordance rate for bipolar-II in identical twins as compared to 31 percent in nonidentical twins. There was a 54 percent concordance rate for depression in identical twins as compared to a 24 percent concordance rate in nonidentical twins. Heritability was 0.77 for bipolar-I, 0.68 for bipolar-II, and 0.38 for major depression (Bertelsen, Harvald, and Hauge). Clearly there are other factors controlling gene expression or there would be 100 percent correlation in these twin studies: if one twin had bipolar disease, their genetically identical sibling would always have it, too. Environmental or epigenetic factors are certainly at work in other aspects of an identical twin's development or physical appearance in that one twin can be slightly taller or stouter than the other or have a mole where the other lacks one. While they may look identical to the casual eye, close friends and family can usually tell twins apart because of subtle differences in their physical appearance or behavior. If these epigenetic factors can alter identical twins' physical appearance or personality, then why not the expression of the genes that trigger bipolar disease?

Adoption studies go a step further to unravel the difference between heredity and environmental influences on mood disorder and bipolar disease in particular. One study showed a 31 percent mood disorder rate in biological parents of bipolar adoptees as compared to a 12 percent rate in the adoptive parents. A control group of non-bipolar adoptees had biological parents with a 2 percent rate of bipolar disease. A group of bipolars who weren't adopted but served as a control group had a 26 percent rate of mood disorder among their biological parents, a result that is very close to the 31 percent mood disorder rate among the biological parents of the bipolar adoptees (Mendlewicz and Rainer). Studies like this strongly suggest a genetic basis for bipolar disease in addition to other factors involved in gene expression.

Genes Implicated in Bipolar Disease

While there have been many studies implicating many different genes as the underlying cause for bipolar disease (Willcutt and McQueen), three of four major studies implicate two specific genes, ANK3 and CACNA1C, that code for proteins involved in the sodium and calcium ion channels in nerve axons in the brain (Barnett and Smoller). This is exciting news, as it implies that bipolar disease may be an ion channel malfunction, much like epilepsy is. Interestingly, both these sodium and calcium channels are made less excitable by lithium in mouse brain studies (Ferreira, O'Donovan, and Meng). Another gene that has been implicated is the DGKH gene, which makes a lithium-sensitive protein in an important biochemical pathway in the brain.

There is another biochemical pathway that is important in regulating our circadian clocks (responsible for our sleep-wake patterns) and three genes interact with this pathway involving the protein GSK3beta. Lithium inhibits the action of this protein, which results in a decrease in the excitability of certain molecules involved in cell death. It also enhances certain neuroprotective factors and serves to regulate the circadian clock (Baum, Akula, and Cabanero). A recently discovered mutation in the CLOCK gene, which in its usual form contributes to normal sleep-wake cycles in humans, produced manic behavior in mice.

The 5-HTF gene has been heavily studied because of its involvement in serotonin transport and the important role serotonin plays in depression. Some studies have shown that a variant of this gene may be associated with bipolar disease, but other studies have shown no connection. Another variant of this gene may be associated with violent behavior, including suicide. The MAOA gene, which encodes for the enzyme that degrades monoamine transmitters, is also of interest because MAOA inhibitors have long been used to treat depression, so there is some connection with mood disorders. There is a mutation of this gene that affects males whose behavior resembles mania with violence and aggression, including suicide. The FAT, or cadherin, gene has also been implicated in bipolar disease, after study of rodent neurodevelopment signaling pathways after administration of lithium or valproate.

An area on chromosome 6 involved in immunity and switching genes off and on has been implicated as having shared susceptibility genes for both bipolar disease and schizophrenia, which could explain how environmental factors can trigger an underlying susceptibility to either disease. This also suggests a common developmental brain malfunction in both diseases (International Schizophrenia Consortium, Purcell, and Wray). Bipolar disease and schizophrenia also share decreased expression of the genes that control myelin production by the special supportive nerve cells in the brain called oligodendrocytes. A more recently implicated gene is neurocan (Ncan), which is thought to be associated with nerve cell adhesion and migration, especially in the areas of the brain involved with emotion, learning, and memory (Cichon, Muhleisen, and Degenhardt).

Bipolar disease therefore appears to be polygenetic, meaning a combination of many different susceptibility genes is likely involved. Each individual gene carries a relatively low risk for the disease on its own but a combination of genes appears to contribute to the manifestation of the disease as well as the unique expression of the disease in each individual. A great deal of research still needs to be done, and is being done, on the specific genetics of bipolar. The polygenetic concept of bipolar is the current theory, just as the single gene concept was in the past; and while it remains unproven, the ongoing genetic research supports this theory at this time.

Your Family Genetics

You may be asking yourself what all of this means for you, your family, and in particular, your children. First, no one can tell you with certainly who will or won't get bipolar disease in your family. There is no prenatal test at this time that can tell you whether your unborn child will develop bipolar disease, nor is there any blood test or brain scan that you or any family member can take to definitively diagnose bipolar disease. The best we can do is tell you the risk of having bipolar based on who in your family has the disease. The more closely related the bipolar person is to you, the higher the risk. If you have bipolar disease, the risk of your child having the disease is around 9 percent. That means that every child born to the family has a 9 percent risk of having bipolar. I've seen some families where all the children develop some form of bipolar spectrum and others where none of the children appear to have it. If you are not bipolar, yet have a first degree bipolar family member, you might still carry the genes and pass them to your children with the same 9 percent risk (Miklowitz 85). If both parents are bipolar or one is bipolar and one has recurrent depression, the risk of having a child with some form of mood disorder, whether bipolar or depression, rises accordingly. If you already have children, all you can do is watch and wait. Early diagnosis and intervention can save years of heartache and suffering and it is becoming more common for teenagers and even young children to be diagnosed with bipolar disease and treated, especially if there is a positive family history.

You may have obvious bipolars in your family tree, but many individuals fail to recognize bipolar spectrum family members. When we grow up around family, we often fail to see them as anything but normal. We accept their personalities without question and our most unusual family members are often fodder for our most cherished family stories. There are certainly a few cases of bipolar disease that appear to come out of nowhere, perhaps from the combination of different susceptibility genes from both sides of the family, and there will always be a few cases resulting from head injuries, birth trauma, or brain diseases such as MS or encephalitis. If you take an objective look at your family, I promise that you will most certainly find your bipolar and bipolar spectrum relatives. Look for suicides, alcoholism or drug abuse, nervous breakdowns, or mental hospitalizations. Those are the more obvious signs of possible bipolar disease. Also look for constant moving and changing jobs or relationships, for long periods of no work or mysterious illnesses, for eating disorders, for reclusive behaviors, or for any eccentric beliefs or actions. Physical or sexual abuse or violence may have occurred, as well as multiple sexual affairs or being constantly in debt or in trouble with the law. If you start collecting stories about past generations of your family, you will most likely find your bipolar ancestors.

I trained with an intern who was pleasant, extremely competent, and hard-working. When he told me he was bipolar, I was skeptical at first, because bipolar disease at that time was usually diagnosed after a major manic attack or suicide attempt. Yet this highly functioning young doctor claiming to have a serious mental illness seemed perfectly normal. He explained that his father, a surgeon, had gotten into trouble for volatile behavior at the hospital where he worked and eventually was diagnosed as bipolar and treated. He recognized the disease in his son by the time the boy was in his teens and sent him to a psychiatrist for official diagnosis and treatment. This young intern was grateful for the early intervention because he didn't have to sacrifice any of his life goals because of the disease. Over the course of a year, I noticed six-month cycles of a mildly elevated mood followed by a mildly depressed mood, but neither cycle was excessive or interfered with this intern's functioning. He and his wife eventually decided to have a child and were not concerned that the disease might be passed down to their baby. They felt confident that they would be just as alert for the disease in their child as the intern's father had been with him. His father's delayed diagnosis had resulted in serious consequences, but his son had an easier time due to early diagnosis and treatment.

What if you are contemplating having children? There are many things that must be considered as you make that decision. Some issues deal with inheritance: bipolar disease, for the most part, tends to "breed true," although your partner may bring additional susceptibility genes into the mix if he has any type of mood disorder or a family history of the same. This may potentially worsen the disease expression in your offspring. For example, families with bipolar-I members tend to continue to produce bipolar-I's, but there can be cross-over, so a bipolar-II family may produce a bipolar-I individual on occasion, and vice versa. Your family may only have the milder forms of bipolar disease but you can't predict when a more malignant variation might pop up in your family tree. Families with bipolar psychosis may occasionally produce a schizophrenic, and vice versa; it appears that the genetic susceptibility to psychosis may be shared between the two illnesses. All families, no matter what type of mood disorder they tend to have, can produce offspring with significant recurrent depression.

The Decision to Have Children

Before you make a decision, you need to look carefully at your own family history and understand that your child may have the worst disease your family could produce or the mildest or no disease at all. That has certainly been true in my own family, where the disease runs the gamut from the mildest form to the most severe, short of suicide. Of course, your child could be normal, but even a normal child might carry the disease and pass it down to future generations. Bipolar disease is not necessarily fatal unless your family is one with multiple suicides, in which case you might view the disease differently than those bipolar families without suicides. Although the disease is treatable, like all chronic diseases, some cases will be more easily treatable than others. The susceptibility to treatment seems to run in families, too. Does your family have the type of bipolar that responds well to medication? Or does it require a number of drugs to reach a shaky equilibrium between stability and mood swings?

Other issues deal with lifestyle; stability must be taken into consideration. Many bipolars are able to lead full, productive, and rich lives. They don't get into trouble, use illicit drugs, drink alcohol to excess, get into financial trouble, or suffer too much, because they have good or even excellent control of their disease. Others, however, may never be completely in control, for a variety of reasons. Having children is a big responsibility and one that is more often than not tiring, frustrating, demanding, and stressful—all the things that can throw an unsteady bipolar completely off balance. If you choose to have children, you will need support during times of instability so that your children will have as stable a life as possible. If you are the breadwinner of the family you will need to give some thought to how your family would survive if you lost your job or had to take a prolonged leave of absence if you became ill, particularly if your family's health insurance is dependent on your job. The stability of your relationship with your partner must also be taken into consideration, as separation or divorce is extremely stressful and even more so if children are involved. If one of your children is bipolar or has some other form of mood disorder, would you be able to handle the added stress and emotional turmoil this would inevitably bring to your life?

If you are a woman, there's always the problem of medication while pregnant. The bipolar medications you are taking when you become pregnant and during pregnancy, or any additional drugs that might be needed during pregnancy should you become symptomatic, should be as safe for the fetus as possible while keeping your bipolar under control. If you are already on a drug that's safe to take during pregnancy, then there's usually no problem. A number of medications used to treat bipolar disease cannot be used during pregnancy and making radical changes in your medication schedule at a time when hormonal changes will already cause some instability is tricky. You'll need a great deal of support during pregnancy and afterward, when you are at risk for moderate to severe postpartum depression or even psychosis. The lack of sleep and disruption of schedule that comes with a new baby in the house has destabilized many a bipolar. Knowing your stressors and having a plan, if you decide to have a child, will hopefully offset problems before they become too large for you to handle. While all the planning in the world can't guarantee a smooth pregnancy and postpartum period, you'll still be ahead of the game if you are as prepared as you can be for bipolar complications.

The Future of Bipolar Genetics

Once the most important susceptibility genes for bipolar disease are found and fully explored, the proteins they code for can be determined, their biochemical actions can be mapped out, and the role they play in bipolar disease completely understood. The proteins these genes code for are likely to be variants of the original "normal" proteins, and these malformed variants will have different actions in their biochemical pathways. Specific drugs may potentially be developed to counteract the altered actions of these variant proteins.

This could mean targeted therapy with increased efficacy and, it is to be hoped, fewer side effects.

In the future, treatment may be person-specific. A bipolar's own suscepti-bility genes may be determined by genetic testing and specific treatment targeting those particular genes and their abnormal proteins may give a level of control that is mainly trial and error today. Perhaps genetic testing can be done at birth so children who inherit the genes for bipolar disease can be watched closely for signs of the disease and treated early. Gene therapy could potentially correct the genetic mutations that cause the variant proteins in the first place or keep the genes permanently turned off so the disease never manifests. Perhaps the "good" of bipolar disease—the genius, creativity, even a bit of the hypomania—could be preserved, while the "bad"—the suicidal impulses, depressions, and psychoses—could be completely eliminated, achieving as close to a cure as possible.

Summary

1. Family studies, including twin and adoption studies, strongly suggest that bipolar disease in inherited.

2. First degree relatives of a bipolar have an increased risk of also developing bipolar disease.

3. If one identical twin is bipolar, the other twin is more likely to also be bipolar, as compared to nonidentical twins.

4. First degree relatives of a bipolar are also at increased risk of developing depression.

5. If one identical twin is bipolar, the other twin has an increased risk of developing depression.

6. Adoption studies show that mood disorders correlate between biological parent and child rather than between adoptive parent and child.

7. There is no single bipolar gene but a group of susceptibility genes that are inherited; much like a poker hand of cards, this mix of genes deter-mines what form of bipolar an individual will inherit.

8. Several genes have been implicated and the most promising appear to alter ion channels in the brain: other suspicious genes are ones that affect the internal body clock, serotonin transport, and myelin production in the brain.

9. The heritability of the disease in each particular family, as well as the dis-ease itself, should be considered when planning a family.

10. When the specific genes that cause bipolar disease are eventually docu-mented, targeted treatment, including gene therapy, may serve to treat an individual's specific set of inherited genes.

Chapter 7

Bipolar Disease in Women

> I firmly believe that this disease fulminates at two distinct life stages: going into puberty and going into menopause. The hormones of youth and the hormones of age. I don't know why men get this. I know why women do.
>
> —Dr. Sis

The Difference Between Men and Women

I don't have to tell you that men and women differ in many ways. One of the biggest differences is that women can conceive and grow and then birth a baby, thanks to an incredibly complex interplay of hormones that begins at puberty and ends at menopause. It's no surprise that these female hormonal fluctuations influence how bipolar disease affects women as compared to men. While men and women suffer bipolar-I in equal numbers, women tend to have more depression than men, thanks to their female hormones, and these depressions tend to be more frequent, persistent, and resistant to treatment. Because of this female tendency toward depression, the spectrum bipolar-II diagnosis is more common in women than men. Even behavior during depressive episodes appears to be gender specific, with women ruminating (about life and loss and whatever they are specifically depressed about), while men tend to be more irritable, aggressive, and actively depressed. Men are usually diagnosed a bit earlier than women because the male presentation is more likely to be manic and a woman is more likely to first be diagnosed with major depression, with a bipolar diagnosis coming later once evidence of mania or hypomania is recognized.

Overall, women tend to have more mixed attacks than men do, display a seasonal variation to their mood episodes, and are more likely to be rapid cyclers. Women are more likely to have other (comorbid) diagnoses such as anxiety, panic attacks, or obsessive compulsive disorder. Cutting is seen in teens and young bipolar women, as are eating disorders and body image problems. And while women can and do have substance abuse problems, men are more likely to self medicate with drugs and alcohol. Additional physical problems are more likely to affect women than men, such as thyroid disease (usually hypothyroidism), obesity, and migraines. These problems are more common in women than men in the general population but bipolar medications or the disease itself exacerbate these conditions in bipolars. The atypical antipsychotics and some of the other bipolar drugs that cause weight gain can cause metabolic syndrome, which results in insulin resistance (leading to elevated blood glucose, which increases the risk for type 2 diabetes), elevated blood lipids, and hypertension. Since women are more prone to obesity than men, they are at higher risk for metabolic syndrome.

The Female Hormones

There are three main sex hormones that control a woman's reproductive functioning. Most of us can name two—estrogen and progesterone—but the third, testosterone, may come as a surprise to many women. Women produce this male hormone just as men produce the female hormone estrogen, just not in the same amounts as men do. This hormone accounts for energy, sex drive, and mood in both men and women. Testosterone levels rise in puberty but vary during the menstrual cycle. Estrogen is an important hormone that affects the female reproductive system in many ways. The estrogen level varies during the menstrual cycle, starting low and building until it peaks near ovulation. If fertilization of an egg occurs and the embryo implants in the uterus, the estrogen level remains high throughout pregnancy; if no pregnancy occurs, the level drops. Progesterone is the hormone that prepares the uterine lining to receive the embryo, so the progesterone peak occurs after the estrogen peak. If the embryo implants in the uterine lining, the progesterone level continues to rise and will be maintained throughout the pregnancy; if no pregnancy occurs, the level will drop and the lining will be shed, causing menstruation.

The rise and fall of hormone levels, as well as the ratio of one hormone to the other, appears to have an effect on mood, particularly depression. Before puberty, depression is equally seen in girls and boys, but after girls begin menarche (their periods), their depression rate suddenly increases over that of boys. Clearly, female hormones seem to play an important role in this increase in depression after the onset of puberty. If you are a woman, you know how mood fluctuates during the menstrual cycle, particularly just before the menses. PMS, or premenstrual syndrome, is characterized by physical and emotional or mood symptoms that occur about 5 days prior to menstruation and then resolve a day or two after menstruation begins. This hormonal condition is very common and occurs in about 80 percent of women. PMDD, or premenstrual dysphoric disorder, is less common, occurring in about 3–8 percent of women, and is a severe form of PMS with marked physical and emotional or mood symptoms that significantly impair functioning and interfere with relationships at home, work, or social settings. Women with bipolar disease, or who have suffered postpartum depression or major depression, or who have a family history of these conditions, are at higher risk of having PMDD. Premenstrual exacerbation, or PME, represents an increase in mood symptoms in association with the menstrual cycle in women with bipolar disease. These women exhibit a more chronic disease course with residual symptoms, a shorter time to relapse, and poorer functioning when compared to women who don't seem to be hormonally sensitive and who recover between mood attacks. It's not known at this time whether PME indicates treatment resistant or incompletely treated bipolar disease (Dias, Lafer, and Russo).

Pregnancy

The decision to have a baby is complicated, for many reasons. First of all, if you are bipolar, you may pass the disease to your child. The chances of that happening aren't high; statistics vary and some studies show a greater chance of inheritance from the father, some from the mother, and some equal; but overall, the chance of your child having bipolar disease if you have it is around 9 percent as discussed in the genetics chapter (Miklowitz 85). Many of the bipolar medications can be harmful to a developing fetus, causing mild to severe anomalies, particularly in the first trimester. Some cause an increase in the risk of miscarriage or stillbirth and others may cause problems in the baby after birth. Going off bipolar medication during pregnancy, particularly in the first trimester, may be one way to decrease risk to the developing fetus; if the pregnancy is unplanned, a woman may not know she is pregnant until she is nearly through her first trimester. If a woman decides to go off bipolar medication during pregnancy, she risks a mood episode that may put her and her baby in more danger than the drug itself would have done. The risk of having a mood episode during pregnancy is quite high due to fluctuating hormone levels. Manic behavior like driving too fast, eating poorly, getting little sleep, missing prenatal doctor appointments, or substance abuse is not good for either mother or baby. Likewise, depression is risky, with sleep and eating disturbances which may lead to a low birth weight baby, premature delivery or complicated delivery requiring C-section or neonatal ICU time or both, not to mention maternal suicide.

A study of mood-stable bipolar women shows the difference between those who terminated medication at conception and those who continued their medication throughout pregnancy. Overall, 71 percent of the women had at least one relapse during pregnancy that was either a depressed or a mixed episode; 47 percent of those episodes were in the first trimester. The women not on medication had a two-fold greater recurrence rate, more than a four-fold shorter median time to their first recurrence, and a five times greater number of ill weeks during their pregnancy (Viguera, Whitfield, and Baldessarini). Even though mood episodes will occur in previously mood-stable, treated women during pregnancy, those episodes will be much worse and more frequent in women who aren't treated. The mental health professional will choose the safest medication for the baby that will also keep the bipolar under as much control as possible, and ideally, only one medication at the lowest dose possible will be used. Once the baby is delivered, the medication can be changed, increased, or added to. Hopefully, the medication will protect from serious postpartum depression.

If you do decide to become pregnant, make sure your bipolar is stable before you get pregnant, then monitor your moods closely during pregnancy and have several people objectively monitor your moods as well. Pregnant women are usually moody, so this may be a challenge for your helpers. You will need to educate them about the specific ways you act and feel when you begin to get hypomanic, manic, or depressed. Work out a treatment plan with your mental health professional that is safe for your baby yet keeps your bipolar under reasonable control, and make sure your obstetrician and mental health professional are working together to care for you. See them both as often as you can get by with (as often as insurance will pay) so they will keep close tabs on your physical and mental health and your baby's health so that problems, should they develop, can be detected and taken care of early.

You will probably require testing in addition to routine fetal ultrasound to look for fetal anomalies if you stay on certain medications; don't be alarmed at this. An alpha-fetoprotein test can be done late in the first trimester and again in the middle trimester to screen for neural tube defects and an amniocentesis test may be needed between 4 and 5 months for further evaluation. Should you develop mania or depression during pregnancy that is resistant to treatment, or you don't want to take additional medication to control your mood state, electroconvulsive therapy (ECT) is a safe option during pregnancy. This sometimes causes uterine contractions which can be managed.

The Postpartum Period

There is increased risk of a mood episode for 6 months after the birth of a baby. While only 15 percent of normal women suffer the "baby blues" three to five days after the birth of a baby, due to the drastic and rapid hormonal shift that occurs, 40–67 percent of bipolar women suffer some degree of depression and a few become psychotic (Miklowitz 266). The mild mood dip in non-bipolar women usually improves within 10 days. Any depression lasting 2 weeks is considered postpartum depression, and women who have suffered depression during their pregnancy are more likely to also suffer a postpartum depression. The immediate postpartum period is tricky, as fluid levels and weight are rapidly shifting, making bipolar medication blood levels difficult to stabilize. Adequate treatment during pregnancy reduces the risk of postpartum depression from 50 percent to 10 percent (Cohen).

The postpartum period carries a high risk of a mood episode because of hormonal shifts, disrupted schedules, the loss of sleep, and the lifestyle changes that occur. Taking care of a newborn baby is exhausting and loss of sleep is a given unless a live-in nanny or an understanding partner or family members help out. If you are a bipolar who can't miss much sleep without triggering a mood episode, you need to think about how you will handle weeks and likely months of interrupted sleep. Breast-feeding is possible, if medication dosing and feeding is timed right, but bottle feeding is less physically taxing on the mother and will allow more sleep since others can help with feedings.

Perimenopause and Menopause

Women with bipolar disease and depression are at increased risk of suffering depression during the transition through perimenopause into menopause, when hormone levels decrease. Specifically, estrogen levels drop and the estrogen/progesterone balance changes drastically. Hormone replacement therapy (HRT) not only helps with the physical symptoms of estrogen withdrawal but may help stabilize the moods that result from this hormonal change. Around 20 percent of bipolar women experience an increase in depression rather than mania during menopause (Miklowitz 276). HRT can help stabilize these women although it can trigger mania and cause rapid cycling in nearly a third of them (Blehar, DePaulo, and Gershon). It can be difficult for some doctors to differentiate mood problems from menopause from worsening of mild or subthreshold bipolar disease:

> Della was a 54-year-old female who had periods of highs and lows throughout her adult life, and while she had never been manic or clinically depressed, she had

mostly been mildly hypomanic with periods of "exhaustion" after these hypo-manic spells. These up and down spells began after the birth of her fourth child when she was 34 but she remained highly functional in spite of them. Della did not have hot flashes, sleep problems, or other typical physical complaints common to menopause, but she became extremely nervous and irritable and couldn't sleep, so her gynecologist started her on HRT. This seemed to work for about six months but the irritability and agitation returned so Della asked her doctor for an increase in hormones. This pattern continued for years and her hormone dose gradually rose over time. If Della forgot her HRT for a few days, she would have a melt-down, once throwing herself on the floor, kicking and screaming like a toddler. Classic bipolar-I symptoms with mania, psychosis, rapid cycling and severe depression eventually developed but Della refused treatment, insisting she simply had a hormonal imbalance. Eventually she was diagnosed with a specific type of breast cancer that is related to the use of high dose HRT and her HRT was terminated at that time. The bipolar continued unabated, with mixed, dys-phoric mood states and suicidal depressions. She remains untreated.

Physical Conditions

Polycystic Ovary Syndrome

Valproate (Depakote) increases the risk of polycystic ovary syndrome (PCOS), where multiple cysts develop in the ovaries and normal ovulation is infrequent or may cease entirely, causing a drop in fertility or infertility. Because of the lack of normal hormonal cycles, these individuals develop endometrial hyperplasia with infrequent, random, and lengthy menstrual periods. Classically, these women have increased testosterone and are overweight, with facial hair and acne. Some women with this condition develop male pattern baldness. They are also at risk for type 2 diabetes and heart disease.

Thyroid Disease

Thyroid disease, particularly hypothyroidism, exacerbates bipolar disease and thyroid hormone (Synthroid is one) helps treat depression even if there is no lab evidence of hypothyroidism. Lithium frequently causes thyroid disease and there is evidence that rapid cycling and hypothyroidism are linked. Women are at increased risk of thyroid disease as they are more likely to have an autoim-mune disease that attacks the thyroid. Most mental health professionals routinely check thyroid function, particularly in patients on lithium, in rapid cyclers, and in women. Dr. Sis was diagnosed with hypothyroidism when we were in college, long before she was diagnosed as bipolar. I could easily tell when she had forgotten to take her thyroid medication from her mood state.

I knew nothing about bipolar at that time, but I knew that her moods and her thyroid function seemed to be intimately connected.

Migraines

Migraines have a lifetime prevalence ranging from 7 to 17 percent, with women more commonly affected due to hormonal factors. Major depression, bipolar disease, panic disorder, and social phobia are found more than twice as often in those suffering from migraines as in those who don't have migraines. Interestingly, there is no association with substance abuse (Jette, Patten, and Williams). Migraine treatment must be coordinated with the bipolar's mental health professional, as some of the current migraine drugs may not work well with the bipolar medications.

Summary

1. Female hormone fluctuations influence how bipolar affects women as compared to men.
2. Due to female hormones, women suffer from depression more than men, and those depressions are more frequent, persistent, and resistant to treatment.
3. Bipolar-II is more common in women than in men.
4. Women are more likely to have mixed attacks, be rapid cyclers, and show seasonal mood variations.
5. Anxiety, panic attacks, obsessive-compulsive disorder, cutting, eating disorders, thyroid disease, migraines, and obesity are more common in women than male bipolars.
6. Overall, the chance of passing bipolar disease to your child is around 9 percent.
7. Many bipolar medications are unsafe for a developing fetus.
8. As many as 71 percent of women have a mood episode during pregnancy and remain at increased risk for 6 months postpartum, with 40–67 percent suffering postpartum depression. Some women become psychotic.
9. Bipolar treatment during pregnancy reduces the incidence of postpartum depression to 10 percent.
10. Menopause causes drastic hormonal changes that can trigger depression; HRT can trigger mania and rapid cycling.

Chapter 8

Why Treat Bipolar Disease?

Like it or not, medication is extremely important in the treatment of bipolar disease and the sooner you come to terms with this, the easier your life will be. While medication is not the only treatment available to you, it is the foundation on which the other treatments are built upon. You have a brain disease that requires medication and all the willpower and self-discipline you can muster won't keep your mood swings under control. If you are lucky enough to possess such skills, use them to follow a good daily schedule and to take your medications on time. Sticking to a daily routine is difficult enough for people who don't suffer from a mood disorder but is extremely hard for those who do. Living a healthy lifestyle and developing a healthy routine is also an important part of your treatment plan and doing so requires a tremendous amount of effort and willpower. Taking pills a few times a day is easy when compared to the work it takes to manage a scheduled, regular daily routine.

If taking pills is so easy, then why do so many bipolar patients resist or sometimes completely refuse to be medicated? If the highs and lows of bipolar disease cause upheaval and sometimes terrible consequences in the lives of bipolars, including failed relationships, financial crises, drug and alcohol abuse, and even suicide attempts, why do bipolars continue to resist and refuse medication that will help even out their mood swings or eliminate them completely? There are many reasons, both physical and psychological, that keep bipolars attached to their disease. There can be unpleasant side effects that many bipolars don't enjoy living with, but these can often be worked around if there is good communication with the prescribing mental health professional. The purpose of treatment may be misunderstood, with many bipolars expecting the depressions to be treated while maintaining the hypomanias, which may not be recognized or accepted as part of their disease. Some simply don't like the idea of having a chronic disease that will require daily medication for life. Many patients diagnosed with a chronic illness feel this way. Others struggle with the idea that they suffer from a mental illness and would rather continue to deny that fact, regardless of the consequences.

Do all bipolars need to be on medication? Is there ever an exception to the rule? There will always be the rare bipolar who has infrequent cycles (decades apart) or who has had a single manic episode without any further mood swings (yet). These individuals may feel that the risks of medication outweigh the benefits in their unique situation and they would rather risk future disease episodes than deal with medication side effects on a daily basis. As long as they have a good support system and start medication immediately if they begin to experience a mood swing, they might get by with not being on maintenance medication if their cycles remain years apart. Unfortunately, some of these infrequent cyclers convince themselves that they have been cured of bipolar disease and they let down their guard, sometimes with disastrous results. No one is ever cured of this disease; given enough time, another cycle usually will occur.

But make no mistake: these infrequent cyclers are rare and you are not likely to be an exception to the rule. Chances are that your cycles are more frequent than once every decade or two, so you might as well get used to the idea that daily medication will be a major part of the management of your bipolar disease. If you feel any resistance to taking medication or have any doubt about why you need to be on medication, I urge you to read this chapter carefully so you can educate yourself on how the brain works and then how it malfunctions in bipolar disease.

The Nervous System

The "Mind"

What exactly is the "mind?" What forms the thoughts, consciousness, memories, feelings, moods, and unique personality that we think of as our "mind?" We know the mind resides in our brain, but where, and how? Our brains are made of nerve cells along with their support cells. There is communication between these cells which form an intricate system of connections linking the various brain regions to each other. The cell to cell communication occurs via charged ions as well as special chemicals called neurotransmitters. Therefore our "minds" are simply the result of electrical and chemical reactions between communicating nerve cells. This can be a difficult concept to grasp, I know. But as simple as this may seem on the cellular level, the connections between nerve cells result in an incredibly complex brain where everything has to be properly connected and working correctly for a person to be "normal" neurologically and psychologically.

When the communication between brain cells become disrupted, the brain begins to malfunction, and the symptoms that develop depend on what part of the brain is affected. Perhaps the nerve cells die, or the connections between nerve cells gets disrupted, or the insulating myelin on the nerve cell axon gets stripped away or the neurotransmitters are out of balance. More specifically, when nerve cells die from lack of blood flow to an area of the brain, a stroke occurs. Connections between nerve cells get disrupted or torn away in severe brain trauma, causing coma and sometimes death. Myelin gets stripped off the axons of nerve cells, causing the nerve impulse to slow down and produces the classic symptoms of MS. A significant drop in the neurotransmitter serotonin can cause depression. All of these conditions are examples of brain dysfunction, and the symptoms, whether physical or mental, vary depending on what part of the brain is affected or how widespread the damage is. Your mood swings are the result of dysfunctional electrical and chemical reactions in the areas of your brain that control your moods. It is important for you to recognize that your abnormally elevated moods (hypomania or mania) are as much a sign of brain dysfunction as your depressions are.

The Central and Peripheral Nervous Systems

The central nervous system (CNS) is made up of the brain and spinal cord. Both receive, interpret and respond to signals from the peripheral nervous system (PNS). The eyes, ears, nose, mouth and tongue send input to the CNS through the cranial nerves, which are also part of the central nervous system. The CNS returns signals as a response to the sensory input it has received from the various sensory sources. The PNS is made up of two types of nerves with two different functions. The sensory nerves send signals from sensory receptors (touch, pain, temperature, proprioception/body position) to the sensory processing centers of the brain, while the motor nerves transmit signals from the brain to muscles, organs, and glands. The exception to this is the reflex arc, where a sensory signal is transmitted to a motor nerve via the spinal cord, bypassing the brain. This allows for prompt action in the face of danger, such as removing a hand quickly from a hot pot without the delay that sending a sensory signal to the brain would require.

Basic Brain Anatomy

Most of the brain is made up of the right and left cerebral hemispheres. These areas, collectively called the cerebrum, are involved in the higher brain functions such as conscious thought, intellect, memory, learning, and speech, and they receive sensory input from both the PNS and the cranial nerves. The cerebrum collects and interprets this sensory information before directing specific voluntary motor action in response to the sensory information it receives. A part of the cerebrum, the limbic system, is involved with emotions and the prefrontal cortex is involved with emotional maturity and inhibition of irrelevant thoughts and inappropriate behaviors. The cerebellum receives sensory information about body position and helps to maintain balance and posture as well as coordinate voluntary body movement, such as walking or climbing stairs. It also assists in learning new motor skills. The brain stem is comprised of the midbrain, the pons, and the medulla oblongata. The midbrain serves as a relay system for the sensory and motor nerve tracts arriving from the spinal cord or exiting from the brain. The pons is involved in breathing and reflex head movements, and the medulla oblongata controls automatic body functions, such as heart rate, blood pressure, digestion, and respiration.

Neurons

A nerve cell is called a neuron, and sensory and motor neurons are slightly different in their structure. A neuron has a cell body, which contains the cell nucleus and the organelles required for cell function, as well as dendrites, which are short, branching arms that extend from the cell body, and either one or two long axons. Dendrites communicate with adjacent neurons by receiving incoming signals from their axons. The axon carries the outgoing signal to the dendrites or the cell membrane or sometimes the axon of adjacent neurons, and is wrapped with insulating myelin which helps transmit the nerve signal (impulse) quickly. An axon sheathed in myelin conducts the nerve impulse at 200 mph, but an axon missing its myelin only conducts at 2 mph. Myelin is produced by oligodendrocytes in the CNS and by Schwann cells in the PNS. The motor neuron has many dendrites and a single axon, while the sensory neuron has axons on both ends of the cell. The CNS also has interneurons that help convey nerve signals between neurons.

The Nerve Impulse

The nerve impulse, called the action potential, travels along the cell membrane and ultimately along the axon and is similar to an electric current. The neuron itself contains potential energy (resting potential), much like a battery contains stored electricity. The neuron is "excitable" in that a certain threshold stimulus will cause a release of that energy. The "resting" neuron is polarized, meaning the outside of its cell membrane is positively charged and the inside is negatively charged. The cell membrane contains many sodium/potassium pumps that keep sodium ions out of the cell and potassium ions inside the cell. A stimulus can reverse these pumps, however, so that positively charged sodium ions rush into the cell, reversing the polarity and making the inside of the axon positively charged. This change in polarity is called depolarization. This reversal of charge that passes along the cell membrane is the action potential that travels until the entire cell membrane has been depolarized. The pumps will eventually restore the normal charge, called repolarization, so that the inside of the cell is once again negative and the outside positive. There is a short delay, called the refractory period, to allow time to repolarize before another action potential (nerve impulse) can once again travel along the cell membrane.

This nerve impulse, or action potential, is a sequential, propagated change in the cell membrane's polarity that travels from the dendrites or nerve cell body down the axon. When it reaches the end of the axon, a chemical is released that travels across the small gap between the axon of one neuron and the dendrites, cell body, or axon of another neuron. The gap that must be crossed is called the synaptic cleft and the chemicals that are stored at the ends of the axons that cross that gap are called neurotransmitters. There are 50 different types of neurotransmitters and the most common are acetylcholine and norepinephrine. Once released, these chemicals diffuse through the fluid in the synaptic cleft and bind to receptors that are specific for that chemical alone. The receptors are on the dendrite of an adjacent neuron, the cell body itself, or another axon. When a neurotransmitter has bound to its receptor, it stimulates depolarization in that neuron's cell membrane: the sodium channels open up, sodium floods the cell, the inside of the cell membrane becomes positive instead of negative, and the action potential passes along that nerve cell's membrane and ultimately its axon to connect with yet another neuron. Neurochemicals have a short lifespan and are either broken down or reabsorbed quickly once they are released from their binding site.

Bipolar Brain Dysfunction

Accumulated Brain Damage

There is a theory that bipolar disorder may be caused by brain cell damage that is accumulated over time as a result of numerous small neurological insults from drug abuse, environment factors, or the body's own steroid production from either acute or chronic stress. Such factors have been shown to be triggers in activating bipolar disease in previously asymptomatic people. It is thought that if enough damage accumulates, a threshold may be reached, triggering the first episode of mania, but continued damage may cause recurrent mania with little or no precipitating factors. This could serve to explain why some people inherit susceptibility genes and never develop the disorder while others do.

Cell Death

The frontal cortex and hippocampus of people with mood disorders, including bipolar disorder, show evidence of cell damage on neuroimaging studies. Because these brain areas help regulate emotion, damage to nerve pathways in these critical brain regions could destabilize moods. Studies of lithium and valproate (Depakote) in rat brains demonstrate an increase in a cell protective protein found in both the frontal cortex and hippocampus, potentially affecting cell survival and preservation of brain tissue in these areas.

Ion Pump Malfunction

Several of the suspect bipolar genes strongly suggest that bipolar may be, at least in part, an ion pump malfunction much like epilepsy, where the neuron resting potential is too low and action potentials are too easy to trigger. In epilepsy, this causes seizures. If the neurons in the parts of the brain that control mood have resting potentials that are too low and their action potentials are too easy to trigger, mood swings could be the result rather than seizures. This would explain why anticonvulsants work as mood stabilizers, as they decrease the excitability of neurons, making it less likely for a nerve impulse to be triggered. Both epilepsy and bipolar disease demonstrate "kindling," where the more attacks a person has, the more attacks she will have in the future. Treatment of both disorders prevents these diseases from worsening over time in the way they would if they were not treated.

Faulty Myelin Production

Examination of brain tissue from bipolar patients after death shows the decreased expression of genes that control production of myelin made by the oligodendrocytes in the brain. Myelin insulates the axons of nerve cells, promoting fast conduction of the action potential along the axon length, just as insulation around an electrical wire allows electricity to flow along the length of a wire without short-circuiting. Likewise, faulty or nonexistent myelin results in "short-circuiting" of the nerve impulses, causing impaired communication between neighboring neurons. This faulty communication may contribute to the abnormal thinking, including delusions and psychosis, that occur in bipolar disease. MRIs show these areas of abnormal myelination in several areas of the brain, but this finding isn't specific for bipolar disease; it can also be seen in patients with schizophrenia as well as other brain disorders.

Neurotransmitters

It is clear the neurotransmitters are involved in some way in bipolar disease, mainly because patients have responded to drugs that cause certain neurotransmitters to stay longer in the synaptic cleft or on their binding sites. Other drugs block release of a neurotransmitter or mimic its action. Glutamate, a neurotransmitter that is excitotoxic at elevated levels, has been found to be increased in the frontal lobes of bipolars and chronic depressives, suggesting that it plays a role in bipolar disease. There is a hypothesis that an increase in epinephrine and norepinephrine causes mania, while a decrease in those neurotransmitters causes depression, based on the observation that the blood pressure drug reserpine, which depletes these neurotransmitters, causes depression. Cocaine, which prevents serotonin, norepinephrine, and dopamine from being taken up in the synaptic cleft, causing all three neurotransmitters to stay around longer, triggers a hypomanic euphoria and can exacerbate mania. Likewise, antidepressant SSRIs (seratonin reuptake inhibitors), L-dopa (dopamine), and tricyclic antidepressants, all of which involve neurotransmitters, can cause mania.

Calcium and Hormonal Influences

Calcium channel blockers have been used to treat mania, which suggests a problem with calcium regulation in the neuron. Valproate (Depakote) increases the activity of a protein that helps regulate calcium in the nerve cell, which may be the mechanism of its neuroprotective activity. Various hormonal disruptions, including hormones involving homeostasis and stress reactions of the adrenals, pituitary, and hypothalamus, are also involved in bipolar disease. Hypothyroidism, including subclinical hypothyroidism, is unusually common in bipolar disease and is always tested for and treated when found. External life stresses in those predisposed to bipolar disease, which stimulates elevated adrenal cortisol levels, or the extreme hormonal changes and stresses of pregnancy, particularly in the postpartum period when psychosis can occur, may precipitate or worsen bipolar disease. Low estrogen levels have been implicated in depression and also in postpartum psychosis, while low testosterone has been implicated in depression in men.

Bipolar Brain Dysfunction Is Treatable

Now you know the basics about how the brain works. You've read some of the theories about what may be going on in the brain with bipolar disease. You can see that they all involve a dysfunction in how the neurons work or communicate with each other, and there is also evidence that neuron death may be occurring. Go back and review the chapter on genetics if you need to remember some of the implicated bipolar genes and what they do in the brain. Everything you had read so far has implicated a structural, physical abnormality as the underlying cause of bipolar disease—neurons that are too twitchy, brain chemicals that aren't at the correct levels, and disrupted neuron communication and connections. Why shouldn't you treat a brain dysfunction if treatment is available? Wouldn't you think it irresponsible if an epileptic chose to live with seizures and refused treatment, especially if that decision was made knowing their disease would get worse if untreated? Bipolar disease appears to be similar to epilepsy, only the symptoms are mood swings rather than seizures. How can you justify not treating your disease when you know it, too, will only get worse if left untreated?

Maintenance Therapy

Maintenance therapy is prophylaxis therapy. I have had migraines since I was 22 and I take a pill every night as prophylaxis to control this inherited, chronic condition. Before I started this treatment, I would have spells of 2 migraines a week, with each migraine lasting 2 to 3 days, for 6 or 8 weeks at a time. I might go 6 months without a migraine and then begin a new cluster. I had some control over my migraines because I knew my triggers, but not everything was controllable. Weather changes were one of my worst triggers and I certainly couldn't control the weather. The flickering of lights was another, as was relaxation. No one wants to be hit with a migraine every weekend or during vacations and most of us are too busy to tolerate losing several days suffering from each one. Since I started prophylactic treatment, I still have the occasional migraine, but they don't happen as often nor are they as severe. When I do have them, I have additional medication I take to treat them. Without my migraine prophylaxis medication, I could never predict when I would lose a day or two or three to a severe migraine. On prophylaxis medication, I wake up in the early hours of the morning with a migraine, I take my rescue medication, and then I sleep off the migraine until it's time to get up. I'm generally functional the rest of the day.

Your maintenance therapy is no different. You will take meds every day so you can live a relatively normal life that isn't interrupted by your illness. You may still have some up-and-down times but the goal of maintenance/prophylactic therapy is to lessen the severity of your disease and to minimize the impact of those times in your life when you do have some mood swings. That means, ideally, that all mood swings stop; but many bipolars will continue to have them, if only in a reduced, occasional, and bearable form that is usually within the range of normal. If you have a more pronounced mood swing on occasion or become symptomatic in other ways, you may need additional medication, just as I sometimes need additional medication to control a migraine that occurs despite the prophylactic therapy.

Many patients ease into maintenance therapy after being treated acutely for mania or depression, so they start out on more meds than they will eventually end up on. If this is your experience, understand that the medications required to control a severe manic attack or a severe depression will probably not be medications you will have to stay on for life. This sort of acute treatment may last anywhere from 6 to 12 months, depending on the severity of your attack. Even after you seem to have recovered, you will be kept on increased medication for another 4–6 months because you are at risk for another attack. Maintenance therapy can begin only when you are fully recovered and out of the danger period for a relapse.

Take Your Diagnosis Seriously

Did you know that up to ⅔ of bipolars have never sought treatment and needlessly suffer every day because of their bipolar? Or that there is at least a 10 year delay before diagnosis in those who do seek help (Goodwin and Jamison II:701)? This allows the disease to worsen over time so that when it is eventually treated, the drugs don't work as well as they would have if diagnosis and treatment had occurred earlier. Unfortunately, about half of bipolars are misdiagnosed as having depression and are treated with antidepressants, which often makes them feel worse and less likely to seek treatment in the future. Sometimes mania can be triggered by the antidepressants. One of my bipolar family members became manic and acutely psychotic 6 weeks after starting an SSRI antidepressant after being diagnosed with bipolar-II rather than bipolar-I. The diagnosis was quickly changed and a mood stabilizer was begun once the psychotic mania occurred. Another family member refuses to report the manias yet continues to seek help for depression while refusing to take antidepressants because of the mixed attacks they cause.

About half of treated patients achieve full remission and the other half relapse within 2 years of an attack. Seventy-five percent of patients relapse within 5 years of treatment and two-thirds of those relapse more than once (Gitlin, Swendsen, and Heller). Clearly, the earlier you get diagnosed and start treatment, the better you will do. Without treatment, your chances of relapsing as well as having a serious relapse are much worse. And while you hope for a full remission, you can never let your guard down regarding relapse.

Whatever bipolar memoir you read or bipolar documentary you see, a pattern of medication noncompliance emerges along with painful and sometimes tragic consequences of that choice of action. Bipolar is a serious mental illness that requires daily medication to control. Surely there are some bipolars who take their medications from the beginning and go back to their lives before their disease so rudely interrupted their flow. Perhaps some aren't quite as functional as they once were as they deal with medication side effects and work on reducing stress and living a more balanced life; but they are contributing members of society, all the same. Where are their memoirs? Their documentaries? In general, they don't write memoirs or star in documentaries because their stories aren't nearly as exciting or compelling as those who have traveled a rockier path. But I know they exist, because one of my family members is among them. A three-week mental hospitalization, caused by a medication change when a serious physical side effect cropped up, left the door open for a cycle that resulted in a severe mixed attack that took a year to recover from. Unfortunately, this was an unavoidable complication of treatment and not a medication noncompliance incident. Still, the consequences were so severe that my family member has no desire to repeat that experience deliberately in the future. This person is a rapid cycler, so the occasional accidental missed pill results in a crying jag at some point in the day that is a reminder the pill has been forgotten. With immediate consequences, it's easy to stay on your meds. Most people, however, do not get such rapid feedback.

Bipolar books containing accounts of madness and multiple mental hospitalizations and—hopefully—wellness in the end, where the individual wises up and finally begins to take their disease and their medication seriously, make for fascinating and inspiring reading. We love an underdog who succeeds in the end. We don't buy books about compliant individuals who take care of themselves right from the start, who go to bed on time, who take their meds, and who maintain their jobs and their relationships. You may feel compelled to read about the severe, uncontrolled bipolars, but wouldn't you really want to be like the other person—the one whose life is in control? Perhaps there's a morbid fascination with reading the account of an out of control bipolar. Is the appeal that you think your bipolar is less severe than theirs or you have more control over your disease than they do? Maybe that's true and maybe it's not. You can only think that way as long as you take medication regularly and keep a good schedule. If you aren't doing those things, you may be in denial. And this is something you are going to have to think about long and hard, because it will interfere with your gaining control of your disease, on many levels.

Andy Behrman, in *Electroboy*, discusses how long it took him to take his disease seriously and to understand how pervasive bipolar disease had been in his life: "I'm coming to understand the impact the manic depression has had on me over the last ten years, informing nearly every poor choice I made, leading me to risk, danger, and trouble. And I'm coming to understand the reality that my manic depression is a chronic condition" (256). Contrast that enlightened understanding of how bipolar disease had affected, and would continue to affect, Behrman's life to Marya Hornbacher's casual, dismissive attitude when finally diagnosed with bipolar disease after a lifetime of mood swings that had worsened to the point where they were occurring on a daily basis: "Bipolar? Kind of an overstatement, but whatever.... Interesting, but not really relevant to me day-to-day—after all, it's not like I'm *sick*" (68). Hornbacher admits that she didn't take her diagnosis seriously for years and the disease continued to worsen. She mistook the manias for her true personality and not as part of her disease. Like so many bipolars, she wanted the medication to control her depressions but not touch her highs, so she took her meds only when depressed, as if the pills would work instantly to cheer her up: "I'll take the meds, though—they'll get rid of the rages, and the afternoon lows. Back to normal in a jiffy, back to my usual *good mood*" (68). The concept of maintenance therapy was something she either didn't understand or didn't want to think about and the consequences were devastating. She worsened to the point where she was hospitalized about every 3 or 4 months for several years, and she wonders what her life would have been like had she taken her disease seriously as soon as she was diagnosed, if she had studied it, thought about it, and accepted it as a part of her life, as it actually had been since she was a child.

Even Kay Jamison, a professor of psychiatry at Johns Hopkins University School of Medicine and one of the leading experts on bipolar disease as well as a bipolar sufferer, went off and on her lithium for years before she finally decided to stay medicated. While she strongly supports medical treatment in her bipolar patients, she had all manner of reasons why she herself was the exception to the rule. When her euphoric hypomanias became increasingly mixed and her cycles worsened, she realized she had to get serious about treatment: "Any temptation that I now have to recapture such moods by altering my medication is quickly hosed down by the cold knowledge that a gentle intensity soon becomes first a frenetic one and then, finally, an uncontrolled insanity ... which would ... rip apart every aspect of my life, relationships, and work that I find most meaningful" (*An Unquiet Mind* 212). As you can see, the most highly functioning bipolars have tried, and failed, to live their lives without medication, and the ones who have succeeded in staying alive and who have found some measure of happiness and success have done so with the help of bipolar medication. Let them share that lesson with you.

Remission Does Not Equal Cure

I know you may have strong feelings about having to be on bipolar medication, and if you don't feel that way now, you probably will at some point in the future. I urge you to discuss your concerns, questions, and fears openly with your mental health professional, especially if you ever begin to think about stopping your medication. Trust me, he has heard it all before. It's common for people to fail to follow instructions, to forget to take a dose, to take too little or too much, or to stop a medication when they are feeling better. This is true for all types of medication, not just bipolar meds, and there is a 50 percent worldwide rate of all types of medication noncompliance (Goodwin and Jamison II: 852). In fact, the first noncompliant bipolar patient was one of the first patients given lithium by Cade, who discovered lithium's anti-manic properties while experimenting on guinea pigs. In this particular case, a chronically and severely manic man had been institutionalized for years, but lithium successfully treated his mania and he was able to go home, only to be hospitalized again in 6 months. His brother told Cade that this man had felt so well he believed he had been cured and didn't need his lithium anymore so he terminated his medication. Six weeks later, he was as manic as he had ever been and right back where he had started (Goodwin and Jamison II:852). Unfortunately, this is a mistake many bipolars make. They assume their disease has magically gone away, when actually the medication is responsible for keeping the disease under control. Take away the medication and the disease will reemerge.

Individuals with chronic diseases such as asthma or diabetes require life-long treatment. Diseases that are relatively well controlled on medication but have periods of relapse are particularly prone to medication noncompliance. If you have heart disease and miss a dose or two, you begin to sicken and quickly become symptomatic, so it's easy to stay motivated to take your pills on a regular basis. But when you take maintenance medication for a relapsing-remitting chronic disease and you feel healthy most of the time, it's easy to forget that the medication is responsible for your health. Skipping a dose or two, or even a week or two of doses, may not result in noticeable symptoms right away. But your physical or mental health is beginning to deteriorate, slowly but surely, even if you don't realize it. The reemergence of symptoms is inevitable, given time. When the attack hits, whether it's an asthma episode or a bipolar mood swing, additional medications or an increase in dosage strength are often needed to treat what could have been avoided by taking the daily maintenance medications. It's always better to prevent an attack than to treat on an emergency basis, and relapses that occur while on maintenance therapy are nearly always milder and easier to treat.

A bipolar on maintenance therapy needs medication most when relapsing into a mood state. During these times the brain isn't working correctly and insight and judgment are often absent, so realization of an impending attack is often lacking. But this is when many bipolars stop their medication. If hypomanic or manic, you may feel so good that you are convinced you don't need your medication, especially if you don't want anything to dampen your high, or you may even deny that you have bipolar disease. If you are depressed, you may not have the energy or ability to keep up with your daily medication schedule, or you may feel so hopeless that you don't see the point of continuing your medications. It is extremely difficult to maintain a regular medication schedule when your thinking changes and your judgment becomes altered. While you may be able to stay on a medication schedule without assistance most of the time, you may need help when you begin a cycle. That is why support and backup from your family and friends are so important.

Hypomania Is Part of the Disease

No doubt you don't like being depressed but you most likely enjoy the increased energy and creativity that comes from being hypomanic, which leads to increased productivity at home or on the job. The temptation to lower your medication dose or fail to report a rising hypomania when you are enjoying an extremely productive, happy period in your life is often very powerful. But this is a temptation you must learn to resist. Terri Cheney explains about monitoring her happiness level: "How could I ever hope to tell a normal person about the terrors of being happy? ... Stop, wait a minute, hold on there—was I happy? ... I had to ask, because what felt like happy now might well be *too* happy in a minute—and we all knew where too happy could lead" (33). For Cheney, being too happy—being manic—usually involved illegal behavior, whether she got caught or not. She monitors her moods in such a way that even genuine periods of happiness are looked upon with suspicion. She calls this "happiness management" (34), which she says has kept her safe from manic attacks but, she feels, has killed much of the joy in her life. I hasten to add that what she has actually "killed" is hypomania and mania, which she both enjoys and fears and therefore struggles to control, rather than normal, non-manic happiness and joy. (When all your happy times have been *too* happy, you lose perspective on what normal happiness and joy are really about.) When the atypical antipsychotic Abilify was added to Cheney's medication schedule, the brakes were suddenly applied when hypomania threatened. Cheney went from being terribly happy to a normal happy, and she eventually learned that happiness wasn't hypomanic excess. She decided the trade-off in stability— the lack of depression, pain, and the consequences of her manic behavior— more than made up for the loss of her hypomanic highs.

The Hypomanic Identity Crisis

It is difficult to know where the disease begins and ends in regard to a bipolar's personality. More often than not, a bipolar will identify with their hypomanic self and feel dulled and "less than" when medicated back to normal, despite the family and friends' relief at having their more-or-less normal loved one back again. You may feel as if the most socially brilliant, fun, true hypomanic or manic version of yourself is the real you and that conviction is understandably hard to let go once the medication brings you down from the hypomanic mountaintop. Andy Behrman contemplates the loss of his hypomanic identity once medicated: "Am I more myself on them or less? There's no sense in trying to determine which me is the real me—in the end, I need the medications if I'm to lead a balanced life. I have a chronic illness, and I can't survive without them" (263). Behrman takes his medications and accepts that he will never be able to stop taking them. He still has mood swings that aren't frequent or severe and are merely an inconvenience he's learned to live with. He understands that he suffers from a chronic physical disease that can be a killer, from suicide or accidental death through risky behaviors while manic, with terrible financial and legal consequences. Like Cheney, Behrman chooses stability over hypomania and mania.

My family member also went through the same identity crisis when clothing, hairstyle, and home decorating tastes, to name only a few things, drastically changed when hypomania disappeared and normalcy once again reigned. If you find yourself going through the same sort of experience, talk honesty with those who knew you before you got sick. They will remind you about who you were before your bipolar disease took control and they will be able to reassure you as you become the person you used to be. Trust them when they tell you that the normal you, rather than the hypomanic you, is the best version of you. Your perception of yourself when hypomanic, no matter how grand you thought you were, is not likely to be accurate.

The Hypomanic Addiction

Kay Jamison also struggled with the issue of who she really was on medication (lithium). When she complained of having less energy and being less lively than she had been before treatment, others would point out that she was now normal, like them. But she bristled at the idea that she should compare herself to anyone but herself: "When I am my present 'normal' self, I am far removed from when I have been my liveliest, most productive, most intense, most outgoing and effervescent.... I am a hard act to follow" (*An Unquiet Mind* 92). She admits to suffering a terrible sense of loss at giving up who she thought she was. She is a mental health professional, but she was in denial that she suffered from an actual disease, although she strongly believes that bipolar is a physical brain disease. She claimed her moods were valid responses to life events, and even though her suicidal depressions nearly cost her life, she still craved her hypomanias and manias, which she likened to an addiction.

Most of Jamison's resistance to her medications was psychological, which is typical, although she suffered significant physical side effects from her lithium in the beginning. Feeling as if she were the exception to the rule, she thought she should be able to control her disease without medication. She also suffered tremendous pressure from a family member for her decision to medicate. As a mental health professional, she knew all the facts. She would medicate during an attack but as soon as she felt normal again she took herself off her meds, time and time again, even as she encouraged her own patients to stay on theirs. She didn't worry about being hypomanic, but as soon as her mood became mixed or manic, she restarted her medication. Eventually she came to realize that she had to make a choice between being crazy and possibly dying from another suicide attempt or being sane and staying alive. She saw that her manias were becoming more mixed than pure, her depressions were deepening and she was becoming more suicidal. She had to face the reality that she wasn't the exception to the rule after all, but it took her a long time to come into compliance with her medication schedule.

Aiming for Normal

You may find that you have forgotten what it's like to be normal. As Jamison said, "But if you have had stars at your feet and the rings of planets through your hands, and are used to sleeping only four or five hours a night and now sleep eight, are used to staying up all night for days or weeks in a row and now cannot, it is a very real adjustment to blend into a three-piece-suit schedule.... I miss Saturn very much" (*An Unquiet Mind* 92–93). Who wants to admit that the real you is less brilliant and creative and certainly less energetic without hypomania fueling the fire? But as much as you'd like to stay on the edge of hypomania, it's dangerous to allow your bipolar to be in control. If you are still cycling, you need to get your cycles under control as much as possible. The more you cycle, the worse your cycles will get over time (kindling). I like to think about this like a path or trail, where you have walked along an area so often that the grass has been flattened and the ground packed down, making travel much easier and faster than when the grass was high and the dirt was soft. The more unmedicated cycles you have, the more you will have in the future and the more intense they will be. Bipolar medication halts, or at least slows down, the cycle schedule and dampens the intensity of the mood swings. While you may never be completely normal, you can aim to be as normal as possible.

All or None

If going off bipolar medication is so common, then why am I making such a big deal out of total compliance? Because terrible things can and do happen when bipolars go off their medications. The problem is that once you get "*too* happy," the consequences of impending mania and the depression that follows, which may be suicidal, never enter a bipolar's mind, especially when hypomanic. All judgment is gone when your brain starts to malfunction in hypomania or mania and you aren't capable of making a rational or healthy decision for yourself. Why take that risk? Too many bipolars take their medication only to stay out of depression or severe mania, while hoping to achieve a hypomanic high. But you can't have hypomania without the rest of the cycles that inevitably follow on its heels. You can't have a pick-and-choose-my-mood attitude toward bipolar control. It's an all or none situation.

Bipolar Medication Side Effects

Side effects can sometimes be burdensome, but this shouldn't be an excuse to terminate your medication. Many side effects disappear in the first couple of months of treatment and those that persist and interfere with your life should be discussed with your mental health professional to see if a change in dosage or the timing of dosage might help. A substitute medication may be needed, as you may have side effects to one drug in a specific category but not to another drug in the same category. Some of the medication side effects are serious, though, and could potentially affect your long-term health. Your mental health professional will be able to guide you on issues regarding bipolar medications and will monitor you for dangerous side effects; that is why you undergo all those blood tests. If a problem shows up, it will be taken care of before it gets too far along.

Keep things in perspective: untreated or poorly treated bipolar disease is serious and can be deadly. There may come a time when you will have to live with a burdensome side effect because the medication is working well to control your disease and there is no alternative medication you can take. Always keep your goal in mind and think about the trade-off—is your side effect worse than the consequences of untreated (and worsening) bipolar disease? My family member suffers an hour of extreme dizziness after the morning medication dose of several medications. This is handled by setting the alarm clock for 5:00 AM, at which time the medication is taken, allowing the next hour for sleeping off the side effects until the alarm goes off again at 6:00 a.m. By that time the dizziness has resolved so that it is safe to shower, and later, drive to work. There are creative solutions to side effects that may at first seem terrible and unlivable. Open, honest communication and trust between you and your mental health professional are necessary if you are going to find the right combination of drugs, in the right doses with the least side effects, that are going to work for your bipolar disease.

Bipolar Self-Medication

If you want to continue to drink or get high but you stop, reduce, or erratically take your meds because of the potential liver toxicity when mixing alcohol or other sedating drugs with some of the bipolar medications, just remember that alcohol and other drugs are a common means of self-medicating bipolar disease. Instead of doing what your real bipolar medications need to be doing, the alcohol and assorted drugs (or even cutting) that individuals use to self-medicate only dampen the mood swings temporarily while destabilizing the mood disorder over the long haul. Carrie Fisher self-medicated with alcohol and codeine, which eventually resulted in an accidental drug overdose: "I used to refer to my drug use as putting the monster in the box. I wanted to be less, so I took more—simple as that.... I just wanted to turn the sound down and smooth all of my sharp corners" (117–18). She used this as an excuse for not taking her bipolar meds on a regular basis. Her thinking was that as long as a drug—any drug—worked, what was the difference? Hornbacher misrepresented her drinking to her psychiatrist, which, along with her erratic medication schedule, resulted in low blood levels of her mood stabilizer. This ultimately caused a severe worsening of her bipolar disease, with multiple mental hospitalizations for quite a few years until she got serious about getting her disease under control. You cannot continue to self-medicate if you expect to control your disease.

Bipolar Stigma

If you feel shame that you have a mental illness, discuss this with your mental health professional and get counseling or talk therapy to help you deal with having a chronic illness. Chronic disease, whether mental or physical, is difficult to accept and learn to live with. If your family members, friends, or faith community don't support you in the choices you've made to treat your bipolar disease then you are going to have a particularly difficult time resisting the pressure of those who should be supporting you in the management of your chronic illness but who may instead try to destabilize you. Some of your friends or family might feel it's a sign of weakness if you take medication to control your moods. Or they might think taking bipolar medication is a different sort of addiction, making one a "prescription addict," which they may feel isn't much different than self-medicating with illicit drugs. Family members might resist the idea that one of their own has a mental illness or a parent might feel guilty, thinking that defective parenting somehow brought on this disease. But bipolar is an inherited disease, therefore it is a family disease. If you have it, others in your family have it as well.

I've found that often the family members who are the most resistant and unsupportive are the ones with some symptoms of bipolar themselves. They feel if they deny that you have it, then they can continue to deny they have it, too. Others simply may not understand bipolar disease and they need to be educated about it. You may never change the opinions of some people and they will continue to perpetuate the stigma of mental illness; don't waste time worrying about them. Spend your energy and time educating those with an open mind who will be supportive of you and who are willing to help you get your disease under control. Our society has become more knowledgeable and accepting of mental illness, particularly depression and bipolar disease, although we still have a long way to go. When you are out in the world as a well-controlled bipolar, you will be shattering the mental illness stigma in the most powerful way possible.

Managing Bipolar Prescriptions

You may struggle with financial restraints such as a lack of insurance or limited insurance mental health coverage, but your mental health provider can help you find ways to afford your medication. You may have trouble getting to the pharmacy, making it difficult to keep your prescriptions filled and current. If you live in a large town or a city with a pharmacy that delivers, getting your prescriptions should be no problem. Some insurance companies encourage the use of a mail-order pharmacy service, so your drugs are delivered via mail. Regardless of how you get your medication, you will need to be vigilant about keeping your prescriptions filled so you don't run out of pills or wait until the last minute to get a refill. Some pharmacies, including the mail-order pharmacies, provide a reminder phone call when it's time to renew a prescription. Refill requests can be done over the phone if you are an established patient. But in the early days of treatment, your mental health professional may want to see you before each refill, so be sure to clarify how refills of medication will be handled. Prescriptions are sent electronically by most doctors, so you don't have to worry about keeping up with that little piece of paper; all you have to do is show up to collect your medications, on time, unless you can get them delivered to you. Pay attention to how many pills you have left in each prescription so you don't run out. You may need help with this at first, if you've never taken medications on a routine basis, but in time it will become a habit that you won't easily forget.

Pregnancy

Many of the bipolar medications are not recommended for use during pregnancy, but some can be used, with caution. If you are a woman and are thinking about becoming pregnant or suspect you are already pregnant, talk to your mental health professional immediately. A change of medication may need to be started quickly, as the fetus is most susceptible to the damage of some drugs in the first trimester. Because of the hormonal changes of pregnancy and the postpartum period, a worsening of bipolar disease may occur. Some women have their first manifestation of bipolar disease during or after pregnancy and postpartum psychosis may occur, so close monitoring is necessary. Getting pregnant or planning to get pregnant is not a good time for coming off bipolar medication on one's own because it is a particularly vulnerable time in a bipolar woman's life.

Summary

1. Bipolar is a serious, chronic, incurable disease.
2. Brain dysfunction causes the symptoms of bipolar disease.
3. Medication is the foundation of bipolar treatment.
4. Many chronic diseases, including bipolar disease, require lifelong medication.
5. The longer the disease remains untreated, the worse it gets and the harder it is to treat.
6. Maintenance therapy is prophylactic therapy.
7. Hope for remission but expect a relapse.
8. Hypomania is part of the disease; your hypomanic self is not the real you.
9. Medication side effects can be handled.
10. Always communicate with your mental health professional about your medication concerns.

Chapter 9

Bipolar Disease Medications

Bipolar disease is a physical brain disease with psychological symptoms, requiring both physical and psychological treatment. The first and most important treatment, at least in the beginning, is medication. Next is some form of talk therapy and last, but certainly not least, is lifestyle management. I like to think of these treatments as the legs of a three-legged stool; all three legs are needed or the stool won't stand up. If any of these three treatments if missing, your bipolar disease won't be completely controlled. This chapter will focus on the first leg of treatment—medication. Chapter 10 will discuss talk therapy and lifestyle management, while chapter 11 will discuss additional therapies, nutritional supplements, and other things you may want or need to do in addition to the three main bipolar treatments.

General Guidelines of Medical Treatment

There is no magic medication formula that works for everyone, as each individual has different symptoms in different degrees of severity and each medication may work a bit differently in each person. Finding just the right medication to get your bipolar under control is a process of trial and error and requires communication and cooperation between you and your mental health professional. It may take up to two years or even longer to find the right combination of medications that work for you. An acute mood attack requires medication that is not needed once you have stabilized. If you were diagnosed during an acute attack, you will eventually be weaned off your acute medications until you are only on maintenance medications. An additional medication or two may be added to your maintenance medication schedule or the dosage of one or more of your maintenance medications may be increased if you begin to get hypomanic or depressed again. The goal of treatment is to stop your cycles completely, but realistically that may not be possible. If your cycles can't be stopped, they can at least be minimized so that you have only muted, infrequent cycles that are far removed from the full-blown cycles of your past. But now and then relapses may occur, particularly in the beginning before an effective treatment plan is worked out.

You must trust your mental health professional to choose the right medication for you, but for that to happen you must be honest about your symptoms as well as your medication side effects. There is no perfect drug or combination of drugs to treat bipolar disease. Many of the drugs have side effects that can range from minor and irritating to truly bothersome or life threatening, so you should approach this trade-off between medication benefits and side effects with an open mind. It's a rare medication, psychiatric or otherwise, that doesn't come with potential side effects, and unless those side effects are unbearable or dangerous, try to tough it out and see if they don't improve or go away in time. Many side effects do, and those that don't can often be treated in order to make them more bearable. Your mental health professional will provide guidance regarding the side effects that are likely to disappear in time and those that are likely to stick around as well as which side effects can successfully be treated by additional medications and which you will need to learn to live with.

Acute or severe mania is treated with antipsychotic medication, particularly the atypical antipsychotics, higher doses of some of the mood stabilizers, and the benzodiazepenes, which are used for their sedative effect until the other antimanic drugs begin to take effect. The most effective drugs are the typical antipsychotic haloperidol (Haldol) and the atypical antipsychotics risperidone (Risperdal) and olanzapine (Zyprexa). Your mental health professional may choose different drugs than these, however. The decision regarding which drug to use with each manic individual is based on the specific symptoms of the mania, such as psychosis, sleeplessness, agitation, aggressiveness, or violence.

Depression is usually treated with atypical antipsychotics, specifically quetiapine (Seroquel), olanzapine (Zyprexa), or with the anticonvulsant lamotrigine (Lamictal). While antidepressants may be used alone for depression if used in the short term, the risk of triggering mania would suggest they are better used in conjunction with a mood stabilizer or other anti-manic drug, although their use in treating bipolar depression is controversial. If an individual is already on a mood stabilizer, adding lamotrigine is the preferred method of treating depression, although some mental health professionals may still add an antidepressant in this clinical situation. If an antidepressant is added, close observation for a switch to mania or a mixed mood state is necessary, although this is less likely when the patient is already on a mood stabilizer. In those individuals who are resistant to all treatments for depression, a single IV dose of an N-methyl-D-aspartate (NMDA) antagonist has shown a rapid reversal of depression. (The NMDA receptor antagonist ketamine is being explored for the acute treatment of bipolar depression.) Maintenance therapy for mood stabilization employs the atypical antipsychotics, lithium, and several epilepsy drugs.

Most drugs are started at low levels and are gradually increased over days and weeks in order to lessen the sedative side effects and to monitor for potentially harmful although unusual or rare physical side effects. The final dosage you end up on may vary widely from another person's dosage of the same drug. If you are on more or less medication than another bipolar, this does not mean your bipolar is more or less severe than theirs. Each person metabolizes (breaks down) each drug at a different rate, and other drugs or substances an individual may be taking can alter the bipolar's blood level of that drug. As other medications or substances are added or dropped over time, changes in your bipolar medication may occasionally be required. Body physiology may change, which can influence the way you respond to your medication, sometimes forcing a change in dose or drug choice. This does not necessarily mean that your bipolar disease is worsening; sometimes a medication "tune-up" is needed because your body has changed its response to your usual medications.

Since many bipolars often end up on several medications to treat various psychiatric symptoms associated with bipolar disease, I am not going to give an exhaustive list of dose ranges, therapeutic levels, or drug interactions; monitoring those numbers and being vigilant for interactions is your mental health professional's job. I will mention over-the-counter medications or substances that might interfere with your bipolar drug, or common antibiotics or other medications your family doctor may give you without realizing those drugs might interfere with your bipolar medication. Your pharmacist should alert you to the possibility of such an interaction to any prescription drug you are combining with your bipolar medication, but if you have any question about what you are taking, feel free to ask your pharmacist or mental health professional for additional information.

I will also mention common as well as unusual or dangerous side effects associated with these drugs, but I don't want to overstate their importance. Most of the side effects mentioned are infrequent, occurring 10 percent of the time or less, although some are more common and percentages are given when available. Many side effects are transient but a few many linger. Some of the side effects are frightening but serious side effects are quite rare and avoiding the remote possibility of having a serious side effect is not a valid reason to refuse treatment. Honest communication between you and your mental health professional and vigilance in keeping your appointments and getting your labs done will allow for early diagnosis and treatment should a serious drug related complication begin to occur. Try to keep this information in perspective, as the consequences of untreated bipolar disease are, in most cases, much worse than the medication side effects that most treated bipolars will have to contend with.

The following medications include the most commonly used drugs in bipolar treatment today. I have tried to include pertinent information for each drug type as well as a representative sampling of drugs within each category. There may be new drugs approved for use in bipolar disease by the time this book is on your library shelf, or one of the commonly used drugs may have fallen out of favor. If your mental health professional is using a drug that's not in this chapter, or is using one in a different way than is described here, chances are there is new evidence to support that treatment. Research in the treatment of bipolar disease never stops. When there is evidence of a potentially more effective bipolar drug, or one with fewer side effects, and your mental health professional thinks you may benefit from that treatment, your medication will likely be changed. The first atypical antipsychotic was a miracle drug for my family member, who was a rapid cycler. Nothing stopped the cycles until that drug was added to the two mood stabilizers my family member was taking, and the improvement was nothing short of a miracle. But if your treatment is working well and you aren't having significant side effects, you will likely remain on the same medication, no matter what new bipolar drug may be available.

When in doubt, ask questions and educate yourself about your medications so you will be fully informed about how your bipolar disease is being treated. Your mental health professional will take good care of you while you go through the process of finding the right medications that work for your bipolar disease. And be patient. Finding the right combination of medications in the right doses takes time and a lot of honest communication between you and your mental health professional. You will need to take your medications on schedule so your blood levels stay steady to allow them to work properly. If the levels are too high you may have increased side effects or toxicity, and if they are too low they won't work to control your moods. But all this hard work will eventually pay off when you begin to get your disease under control.

The Medications

Lithium Carbonate (Duralith, Eskalith, Eskalith-CR, Lithobid, Camcolit, Priadel)

HISTORY OF LITHIUM TREATMENT

In the past, people afflicted with chronic illnesses were attracted to mineral springs, believing that soaking in or drinking the mineral waters would restore health and vitality. Even as early as the second century AD, Galen advised patients suffering from mania to drink mineral water, some of which apparently contained high concentrations of lithium. Episodic depression was treated with lithium in the 1880s, but because there was no proven efficacy at that time, its use was eventually discontinued.

The first documented clinical use of lithium salts for treatment of bipolar disorder was described in 1949 by an Australian psychiatrist named Dr. John Cade, who was injecting urine from mentally ill patients into guinea pigs in an attempt to reproduce psychiatric symptoms. Unfortunately, guinea pigs injected with the urine of the mentally ill died faster than control guinea pigs injected with the urine of the non-mentally ill. Cade knew that uric acid was psychoactive because it stimulated neurons, so he suspected that high levels of uric acid was present in the urine of the mentally ill patients and might be responsible for these guinea pig deaths. He added lithium to the urine of the mentally ill to increase the solubility of the uric acid and then injected this lithium urate-urine solution into his guinea pigs. He was surprised to find those guinea pigs very calm and less responsive to stimuli, as if they had been mildly sedated.

After a careful series of controlled experiments, Cade isolated the sedative effects to the lithium. This led him to give lithium to ten of his manic patients who responded in much the same way as the guinea pigs had. In fact, some of his patients became well enough to leave the hospital and return to their homes after years of being institutionalized. Unfortunately, Cade's paper in the *Medical Journal of Australia* did not revolutionize the treatment of bipolar disease as it should have. The 1940s had seen lithium salt used as a sodium salt substitute for those with heart disease or hypertension, with the unexpected result of serious lithium toxicity that sometimes resulted in death. No one was eager to embrace this "poison" as a drug, no matter how miraculous its effects might be.

Danish physician Mogens Schou was intrigued by Cade's paper, however, and confirmed the anti-manic findings in his own study. Later, he would show that lithium also reduced bipolar cycling and recurrent depressions. Schou worked patiently to get lithium accepted by the psychiatric community, but he was criticized by those who refused to believe in lithium's efficacy despite having never tried the drug on their own patients. Since lithium is a naturally occurring substance (one of the periodic table elements), Schou had difficulty funding his research since a natural element couldn't be patented, and without the lure of profit, no drug company had a commercial interest in developing a drug that was a simple, elemental compound. Schou's tireless efforts and impeccable research, along with the contributions of several other researchers, eventually paid off, however. Lithium carbonate was approved by the Food and Drug Administration (FDA) in 1970 for the treatment of mania and was approved for preventative and maintenance therapy for manic depression in 1974. It is still the most commonly used drug for acute mania and mood stabilization and maintenance, especially for bipolar-I disease.

LITHIUM IN BIPOLAR TREATMENT

Lithium appears effective in treating all mood states, including depression and the mixed mood state, but it works best for the classic bipolar-I pattern of manic highs and depressed lows. It also decreases the frequency and severity of mood cycles, is thought to be neuroprotective, and appears to have an anti-suicide effect, decreasing the risk of suicide by almost 10 times what it would be without the drug. Since lithium is an element it cannot be metabolized by the body; when it is excreted by the kidneys, it is unchanged. The half-life of lithium, which is defined as the amount of time it takes for half a dose to be excreted from the body, is variable, depending on an individual's age and kidney function. This can range from a half day to a day and a half. It takes time for lithium to begin to work—from a week and a half to two weeks to treat acute mania and 6 weeks or longer to interrupt cycling. Faster acting drugs are often added to lithium to treat acute mania but these drugs may be removed once stability is achieved.

Blood tests performed prior to beginning lithium therapy measure electrolytes, thyroid and renal function, the complete blood count, and whether a woman is pregnant or not if she is of childbearing age. During treatment, renal and thyroid function and lithium levels are routinely monitored. Liver function tests are also needed if lithium is taken with valproate. Nausea is a common complaint, so lithium should be taken with food, although this side effect usually improves with time. The delayed absorption lithium preparations have less GI side effects. There may be excessive thirst and increased urination, and diarrhea may also occur. If increased urination and thirst are excessive or extreme, this may indicate a condition known as diabetes insipidus. In this condition, the kidneys are unable to reabsorb fluid, causing excessive urination, which in turn leads to excessive thirst in an attempt to replace the fluid that is lost due to excessive urination. Tremor, flaring of skin conditions already present, and weight gain are other common side effects. Sometimes swelling of the extremities may occur. Hypothyroidism is quite common and requires treatment.

Because of lithium's potential toxicity, blood levels must be closely monitored and good renal function and adequate hydration are required in order to prevent toxicity. Symptoms of toxicity include worsening of baseline side effects, such as tremor, or an upset stomach that has progressed to vomiting and diarrhea. More pronounced symptoms of toxicity include a staggering, drunken gait, slurred speech, light-headedness or faintness, confusion, and giddiness. Toxicity is a medical emergency and can lead to coma and death. Sometimes toxicity can occur even at therapeutic blood levels with electrolyte disturbance, so anything causing sodium loss, such as a diuretic use, or nausea, vomiting, or dehydration, must be avoided. Toxicity after heavy sweating has been reported but has not been confirmed as a true cause of toxicity. Changes in salt intake, whether increased or decreased, should also be avoided, as this can cause either decreased blood levels of lithium (in increased salt intake) or elevated blood levels of lithium (in decreased salt intake), resulting in toxicity.

NSAIDs (ibuprofen, naproxen, etc.) should be taken with caution because they can increase lithium levels, but aspirin and acetaminophen (such as Tylenol) can be safely taken. The ACE inhibitor category of blood pressure medication (captopril, lisinipril, ramipril, etc.) or the calcium channel blocker category (diltiazem, verapamil) may also raise lithium levels, along with some antibiotics (tetracycline, doxycycline), the seizure drug phenytoin (Dilantin), metronidazole (Flagyl), and especially methyldopa (Aldomet), which can cause toxicity at normal lithium levels. Drugs that may lower lithium levels include the asthma drug theophylline, acetazolamide (Diamox), and caffeine. If you are on lithium and are drinking caffeine on a daily basis, stopping all caffeine abruptly will cause your lithium levels to rise.

Anticonvulsants

These epilepsy medications, often prescribed "off label," tend to be used in the younger population and in rapid cyclers, as they work better than lithium for this group of individuals. Antidepressants are often avoided in these patients because their use may trigger mania, but fortunately lamotrigine (Lamictal) has been proven to be helpful in treating depression. The most commonly used anticonvulsants are carbamazepine (Tegretol), divalproex sodium (Depakote), and lamotrigine (Lamictal), but topiramate (Topamax) and oxcarbazepine (Trileptal) are becoming more widely used.

CARBAMAZEPINE (TEGRETOL, EQUETRO)

This drug is used for mood stabilization and for treating mania and mixed attacks but is not a first-line drug when treating bipolar disease because of the side effects it produces, including serious bone marrow toxicity (aplastic anemia or agranulocytosis). This is more likely to happen if the drug is given with the atypical antipsychotic clozapine (Clozaril). Although this complication is rare, the blood count must be monitored and excessive bruising or frequent infections should be promptly reported. Carbamazepine works well on lithium resistant individuals as well as rapid cyclers, so it still has a place in bipolar treatment.

Sleepiness and dizziness are common during initial dosing, and driving or engaging in other behavior that requires quick reflexes is discouraged until these early side effects disappear. Nausea, constipation, memory problems, blurred vision, and muscle coordination problems may also occur. Fortunately, some of these side effects diminish with time. Very rarely, liver failure, pancreatitis, electrolyte disruptions, blood abnormalities, and rashes such as Stevens-Johnson syndrome may occur. Stevens-Johnson syndrome is a life threatening condition where the skin cells die and the epidermis, or outer layer of the skin, separates from the dermis, or inner layer of the skin, beginning with the mucous membranes (usually the mouth and lips) and spreads to the face and then the skin of the body.

Alcohol or other sedative medications should not be taken with carbamazepine because the sedative side effects will be cumulative. This drug has a slow and unpredictable GI absorption pattern with a long half-life (anywhere from 25 to 65 hours) that decreases over time because the drug stimulates the liver to increase its metabolism, along with other drugs, including birth control pills. Because of this accelerated liver metabolism, women may not be protected from an unplanned pregnancy if birth control pills are their only form of contraception. Carbamazepine also decreases the levels of the asthma drug theophylline, thyroid hormones, and corticosteroids, but it may increase levels of the calcium channel blocker/antihypertensive drugs diltiazem (Cardizem) and verapamil (Calan). Cimetidine (Tagamet), the antibiotic erythromycin, the antibiotic/tuberculosis drug isoniazid, grapefruit juice, and the influenza vaccine may increase carbamazepine blood levels. This drug should not be given if liver disease, cardiovascular disease, or bone marrow abnormalities are present.

OXCARBAZEPINE (TRILEPTAL)

This drug is similar to carbamazepine but with an improved side effect profile and no bone marrow suppression. It can decrease sodium levels, which can present as ankle swelling, fatigue, and a flu-like feeling. Stevens-Johnson syndrome is a rare side effect, as it is with carbamazepine. The same drug interactions and warnings listed for carbamazepine are valid for this drug, too. Metabolism is through the liver, although the product of this drug breakdown appears to actually be the effective, active form of the drug rather than the original form, so good liver function is important. The half-life of both the drug and the breakdown product is 19 hours. As with carbamazepine, birth control pills are broken down at an accelerated rate with its use, raising the risk of unplanned pregnancy.

Valproate Sodium/Valproic Acid/Divalproex Sodium (Depakene, Depakote, Depakote ER, Stavzor)

This drug was approved in 1995 for the treatment of acute mania in bipolar-I and although it has never received approval for use as a maintenance drug for mood stabilization, it is commonly used "off label" for treatment. Valproate can be combined with lithium if necessary and is effective in rapid cyclers and those with mixed mood episodes. The dose can be raised quicker than lithium and it works faster, too, so it is useful in treating an acute mixed or manic attack and it has a better side effect profile than lithium. This drug is metabolized through the liver with a half life ranging from 9 to 16 hours. Blood tests prior to treatment include liver function, a lipid profile, a complete blood count, and electrolytes, as well as a pregnancy test in women of childbearing age. Monitoring during treatment includes drug levels, liver function, electrolytes, blood counts, and a fasting blood sugar level if weight gain is excessive or diabetes is suspected.

Common side effects include the GI complaints of an upset stomach, nausea, or diarrhea, although the divalproex sodium form of the drug appears to cause less GI irritation. Nervous system complaints include sleepiness, nervousness, insomnia, tremor, and dizziness, along with blurred vision. There are also reports of muscle aches, hair loss, elevated liver enzymes and, rarely, liver failure. Severe pancreatitis can also occur, which may become hemorrhagic and can sometimes be fatal, although this is very rare. A decrease in platelets or an elevation in blood ammonia levels may occur. This drug may cause a false positive urine ketone test.

Sedating drugs combined with valproate lead to increased drowsiness, therefore painkillers containing opiates, benzodiazepines, sedating antidepressants and antipsychotics, alcohol, antihistamines, and over the counter herbal medications such as St. John's wort and valerian root should be taken with caution. There is an increased risk of bleeding when valproate acid is taken with the NSAIDs, drugs containing aspirin, blood thinning drugs like warfarin (Coumadin), willow bark, and valerian. Cimetidine (Tagamet), salicylates (aspirin-containing products), and the antibiotic erythromycin may increase this drug's toxicity, while the antibiotic/tuberculosis drug rifampin can lower blood levels. If this drug is taken with carbamazepine, the blood levels of carbamazepine may vary and seizure control may diminish if the carbamazepine is taken for epilepsy. If valproate is given with lamotrigine (Lamictal), the risk of developing Stevens-Johnson syndrome is increased.

Lamotrigine (Lamictal, Lamictal ODT)

This drug is effective in treating the depressed phase of bipolar and when used for maintenance it lengthens the time between cycles. Lamotrigine is readily absorbed in the GI tract and has a half-life of just over 24 hours although this may be increased or decreased when other drugs are added. Because this drug is broken down in the liver and excreted by the kidneys, good liver and kidney function is required. Acetaminophen (Tylenol) causes the kidneys to clear the drug from the body faster, resulting in lower blood levels, while valproate raises blood levels. There is a risk of developing an allergic rash or hives, including Stevens-Johnson syndrome, particularly when taken with valproate, so slow dosing is recommended, which seems to make these complications less likely.

GI complaints such as nausea, vomiting, abdominal pain and constipation and other side effects such as runny nose, cough, sore throat, dry mouth, back pain, tiredness, and insomnia occur but are usually mild and disappear with time. Significant but infrequent side effects include sedation, dizziness, nystagmus (eyes flicking back and forth), diplopia (double vision), and ataxia (poor balance, with a staggering walk). Although tardive dyskinesia—which is a condition involving purposeless, involuntary physical movements like lip smacking, tongue thrusting, or chewing but can involve limb or trunk movement—is usually associated with the antipsychotics, it is a rare side effect with this medication. While tardive dyskinesia may be permanent once it begins, it is usually confined to the mouth area, is relatively minor, and doesn't worsen over time, although it may temporarily worsen with stress. Akathisia, defined as an overbearing and very unpleasant feeling of motor restlessness that forces an individual to get up and move, may also occur.

Antipsychotics

Traditionally, antipsychotics (also called major tranquilizers or neuroleptics) were used to treat psychosis (disordered thinking, delusions, or hallucinations), but they are used in bipolar disease to rapidly treat manic or mixed mood states, regardless of whether psychosis is present. The two categories of antipsychotics are the typical and atypical antipsychotics. The typical antipsychotics are older drugs, such as Thorazine (discovered in the early 1950s), while the atypical antipsychotics are newer drugs and work on the brain in a different way and have different side effects than the older, typical antipsychotics. The typical antipsychotics are absorbed well, although absorption is affected by both food and antacids. They work rapidly, reaching peak levels anywhere from 30 minutes to 5 hours after ingestion, with an average peak of 3 hours, and a steady state blood level occurs at around 3 to 6 days, with a half life of 3 to 27 hours. These drugs are mostly metabolized in the liver but some metabolism occurs in the intestinal wall. The atypical antipsychotics are well absorbed with or without food, with the exception of ziprasidone (Geodon, Zeldox), which is better absorbed when taken with food.

These drugs quickly sedate psychotic or extremely manic patients, but it takes weeks for the antipsychotic effect to occur. Bipolar depression, particularly if combined with psychosis, can be treated with these drugs, particularly quetiapine (Seroquel) and Symbyax (fluoxetine/olanzapine or Prozac/Zyprexa). The typical antipsychotics are more likely to cause tardive dyskinesia and other extrapyramidal symptoms, while the atypicals are more likely to cause metabolic syndrome with a rise in blood lipids, blood sugar (causing type 2 diabetes), and weight gain (particularly in the belly) that increase the risk for cardiovascular disease and cerebrovascular events. Elevated blood sugar can be severe enough to cause ketoacidosis, coma, and death.

Neuroleptic malignant syndrome (NMS), a life threatening condition with symptoms of muscle rigidity (akin to rigor mortis), fever, and autonomic instability (unstable vital signs), may occur with the atypical antipsychotics. This syndrome starts with cramps or tremors, and a fast, irregular heartbeat; the sufferer may also become confused or succumb to sweaty shock. Eventually the muscle cells begin to die and urine production decreases. Unfortunately, these symptoms may sometimes be confused with a psychiatric catatonic state. Early diagnosis is critical, as this condition is a life threatening medical emergency. Supportive care while withdrawing the medication is the only treatment.

Tardive dyskinesia occurs in about 5 percent of people per year and the longer an individual is on an antipsychotic, the more likely this side effect will develop. As mentioned above, it is more commonly caused by the typical rather than the atypical antipsychotics and it appears that one atypical antipsychotic, clozapine (Clozaril), may not cause tardive dyskinesia, although this hasn't yet been fully proven. (Clozapine is being used in schizophrenia but hasn't been approved for use in bipolar disease.) There is no definitive treatment for tardive dyskinesia at this time. If an individual develops this side effect and the antipsychotic medication is stopped, the tardive dyskinesia may decrease or go away, it may remain unchanged, or it may worsen (this is called "unmasked tardive dyskinesia").

Extrapyramidal side effects (with the exception of tardive dyskinesia), which can occur rapidly, especially in young people who have never been on an antipsychotic, are nearly always reversible. Terminating the drug will usually eliminate this side effect. There are many ways extrapyramidal side effects may present. Symptoms of Parkinson's may be present, such as a shuffling gait, rigidity of the arms and legs, tremor, and a mask-like facial expression. Akathisia, the feeling of motor restlessness, may occur and this can be treated with beta blocker medication. Muscle spasms of the neck, called torticollis, are painful and may be debilitating; the muscles that move the eyes may spasm, rolling the eyes upward; or various other muscles in the body may spasm and cause difficulties. Anticholinergic treatment, in either pill or injectable form, is available to decrease these muscle spasms and other Parkinsonian symptoms. The injectable form works rapidly, while the pills are used for ongoing treatment. There are side effects to these drugs, however, such as dry mouth or dry eyes (which may cause blurred vision), urinary retention, or constipation. Sedation or even confusion and delirium may sometimes occur, particularly when added to other, sedating psychiatric medications. The antipsychotics with the greatest risk of extrapyramidal symptoms, like Haldol, have fewer anticholinergic side effects and less sedation. The antipsychotics with less risk of extrapyramidal side effects, like Thorazine), have more sedation and anticholinergic side effects.

Atypical Antipsychotics

ASENAPINE (SAPHRIS)

This drug is usually given with lithium or valproate but may be used alone in the treatment of acute mania or mixed states. It is usually taken twice a day. This sublingual (under the tongue) medication should be carefully removed from its packaging by peeling off the foil (not pushing the pill through the foil) and handled by dry, not wet, fingers. When placed under the tongue, the medication will dissolve in the saliva and should not be chewed, crushed or swallowed. Nothing should be taken by mouth for 10 minutes after taking this medication to allow for continued oral absorption. Tingling or numbness of the mouth may occur after taking this medication but this usually goes away within an hour. Oral irritation, blisters, or ulcers may rarely occur.

Combining this drug with another drug that prolongs the heart's QTc interval may cause a fatal arrhythmia. Drugs such as quinidine, quinine, or procainamide, amiodarone (Nexterone) or sotalol (Betapace/Sotalex), the antibiotics erythromycin, azithromycin (Zithromax), and ciprofloxacin (Cipro), or several other antipsychotics that also prolong the QTc interval should be avoided. Likewise, low levels of potassium and magnesium in the blood increase the risk of QT prolongation, as do diuretics, severe sweating, diarrhea, or vomiting. Using alcohol while taking this drug may cause toxicity. Other drugs or substances that may interact are aspirin, codeine, cimetidine (Tagamet), insulin, metformin, oxycodone, hydrocodone, some antifungal medications, alpha blockers, antispasmodics (like atropine or scopolamine), drugs that cause drowsiness (antihistamines and other allergy or cough and cold medications), sleep or anxiety drugs, muscle relaxants, and nicotine (smoking). Drugs that may increase the risk of seizure when combined with asenapine are theophylline (asthma drug), tramadol (a non-narcotic pain reliever), and tricyclic antidepressants.

Common side effects include dizziness (11 percent), drowsiness (24 percent) and headache (12 percent). Low blood pressure may result in lightheadedness if rising quickly from a seated position or from lying down; moving slowly will decrease this side effect. Tardive dyskinesia or extrapyramidal symptoms may occur in 7 percent (excluding restlessness) and should be reported to your mental health professional immediately. These symptoms include akathisia, anxiety, agitation, nervousness, drooling, difficulty swallowing, stiff muscles, muscle spasms or cramps, a shuffling walk, and a mask-like facial expression. Hyperglycemia may result in weight gain in 5 percent and worsen preexisting diabetes or trigger new-onset diabetes. If you are not diabetic, report any significant increase in thirst or urination to your mental health professional so you can be tested for diabetes.

This drug may increase prolactin levels (the hormone that stimulates milk production). In females, an increase in prolactin may result in the production of breast milk and may cause irregular periods or even stop periods completely. Men may suffer a decrease in sexual ability, may become unable to produce sperm, or develop gynecomastia (enlarged breasts). These side effects should be immediately reported to your mental health professional. Elevated prolactin levels (hyperprolactinemia), if used long term and associated with decreased gonadal function, may lead to osteopenia or osteoporosis in both sexes. Bone marrow problems also occur with this drug, presenting as chronic or acute infection, so fever or a persistent sore throat or any symptoms suspicious for infection should be immediately reported. Seizures, severe dizziness, fainting, and any sort of heart arrhythmia should also be reported. This drug can cause neuroleptic malignant syndrome. Finally, an allergic reaction is always possible, so rash, hives, swelling of the face, tongue, and throat, and trouble breathing should also be reported.

Quetiapine (Seroquel, Seroquel XR)

This drug is used to treat acute mania or depression and can be used alone or with lithium or divalproex. It is usually taken once a day, in the evening, without food or with a light meal and swallowed whole (do not chew or crush or split it unless the pill is scored and you have been given permission to do so). Interactions occur with a large number of drugs, including those which cause a prolonged QTc interval in the heart. An abbreviated list of suspect drugs or other substances that may cause unfavorable interactions are cimetidine (Tagamet), the antibiotics erythromycin, azithromycin, ciprofloxacin (Cipro), and clarithromycin (Biaxin), certain antifungal medications, albuterol (asthma inhaler), caffeine, ephedrine, epinephrine, quinine, ethanol, insulin, steroids, eucalyptus, grapefruit, marijuana, melatonin, metformin, methadone, methamphetamine, morphine, opium, oxycodone, tramadol, henbane, and St.

John's wort. This drug can cause a false positive drug screen test for methadone or tricyclic antidepressants.

Common side effects (greater than 10 percent) include headache, dry mouth, dizziness, constipation, upset stomach, blurred vision, and sleepiness. Moving slowly when getting up from a seated or prone position should help with dizziness. This drug may worsen preexisting hypotensive conditions, blood lipids may increase, and hyperglycemia and weight gain may occur, with possible diabetes and ketoacidosis as complications. Extrapyramidal symptoms, neuroleptic malignant syndrome, and tardive dyskinesia may occur. Men may have erections lasting 4 or more hours (priapism); if this happens, get help right away to avoid permanent problems. This drug may also cause hypothyroidism, liver dysfunction, heart palpitations, cardiomyopathy, galactorrhea (milk production), Stevens-Johnson syndrome, hyponatremia (low sodium), somnambulism (sleep walking) and a low white count as well as hypersensitivity including life threatening anaphylaxis (an allergic reaction).

Ziprasidone (Geodon, Zeldox)

This drug is used to treat acute mania and mixed attacks but is sometimes used as a mood stabilizer in conjunction with lithium or valproate. It is usually taken twice daily with food. Blood glucose should be monitored in those at high risk for diabetes, as hyperglycemia may cause ketoacidosis and death. Elevated prolactin levels may also occur. As always, monitoring the blood closely for the first few months of therapy is important to make sure the white count remains normal. This drug increases susceptibility to heat stroke, so it is important to avoid getting overheated. Hot tubs should be avoided.

This drug prolongs the QTc interval and should not be combined with any drug that does the same, and the drug interactions are similar to those listed under the atypical antipsychotic quetiapine (Seroquel). Common side effects include sleepiness (15 percent) and headache (11 percent). Side effects that occur less than 10 percent of the time include cough, constipation or diarrhea, nausea or anorexia, dyspepsia, extrapyramidal symptoms (including restlessness or tardive dyskinesia), hypotension, rash, muscle aches, runny nose, or a rapid heartbeat. Unusual side effects, occurring less than 1 percent of the time, include seizures or fainting, increased prolactin levels, neuroleptic malignant syndrome, allergy, and priapism.

Risperidone (Risperdal, Risperdal Consta, Risperdal M-Tab)

This drug is used in the treatment of acute mania or mixed attacks and may be used in conjunction with lithium or valproate. It is taken once or twice a day, with or without food. If used in liquid form, the dose can be placed in 3 to 4 ounces of water, coffee, orange juice, or low-fat milk (not cola or tea), but it has to be mixed immediately before the dose is taken and not prepared in advance. Since this drug also prolongs the QTc heart interval, the same drug contraindications apply as with quetiapine (Seroquel). Pseudoephedrine use should be monitored closely.

Sleepiness is seen in up to 45 percent, insomnia in up to 30 percent, and agitation in up to 25 percent. Anxiety, headache and a runny nose occur in 15 percent and the typical GI side effects in less than 10 percent. An aggressive reaction, dizziness, extrapyramidal symptoms, rashes, a rapid heartbeat, and gynecomastia in children can occur in up to 5 percent. Hypotension, elevated blood lipids, ketoacidosis from hyperglycemia/diabetes, bone marrow problems including a low white cell count, delirium, and seizures are seen in less than 1 percent. Rare side effects include hyperthermia or hypothermia, neuroleptic malignant syndrome, priapism, thrombotic thrombocytopenic purpura (TTP), sleep apnea, and urinary retention. An increased incidence of cardiovascular disease has been reported with this drug.

Aripiprazole (Abilify, Abilify Discmelt)

This drug is used in the treatment of acute mania or mixed attacks and may be used with lithium or valproate. This drug comes in liquid form (stored cold) that can be taken with or without food, or as a disintegrating oral tablet that dissolves in the mouth. The drug interactions and precautions are the same as the other atypical antipsychotics. Weight gain is reported in up to 30 percent, headache in up to 27 percent, agitation in up to 19 percent, insomnia in 18 percent, anxiety in 17 percent, nausea and vomiting in 15 percent, akathisia in 13 percent, and lightheadedness and constipation in 11 percent. Side effects that occur in less than 10 percent include dizziness (10 percent), dyspepsia (9 percent), sleepiness (8 percent), fatigue, restlessness, and tremor (6 percent), dry mouth, extra pyramidal disorder, hypotension (5 percent), and muscle stiffness (4 percent). Other side effects include abdominal discomfort, blurred vision, cough, pain, rash, and a runny nose. Side effects that occur in less than 1 percent include muscle rigidity, altered mental status, dysphagia, increased body temperature, autonomic instability, neuroleptic malignant syndrome, seizure, and tardive dyskinesia. As with all the atypical antipsychotics, a low white count, hyperglycemia, elevated blood lipids, and hypotension may occur.

Olanzapine (Zyprexa, Zyprexa Relprevv, Zyprexa Zydis)

This drug is used in the treatment of acute mania or mixed attacks and may be used in conjunction with lithium or valproate. It is taken once a day, with or without food. The list of drug interactions is the same as the other atypical antipsychotics. Up to 40 percent experience weight gain, depending on the dose, around 39 percent have elevated triglycerides, and another 39 percent have elevated cholesterol. Sleepiness, also dose dependent, is seen in up to 39 percent. Increased prolactin levels are seen in 30 percent, elevation of the liver enzyme alanine aminotransferase (ALT) can be seen in up to 12 percent, and constipation and dyspepsia in 11 percent. Extrapyramidal symptoms and tardive dyskinesia, dose dependent again, are seen in 15–32 percent, dry mouth in up to 22 percent, weakness in 20 percent, dizziness in 18 percent, and accidental injury and insomnia in 12 percent. There is an increased risk of hyperglycemia and diabetic ketoacidosis, hyperosmolar coma, or death (less than 1 percent). Orthostatic hypotension (dizziness or fainting when rising from a seated or prone position), narrow angle glaucoma, prostatic hypertrophy, acute hemorrhagic pancreatitis, venous clots and pulmonary embolus, suicidal intent, and stroke may also occur.

OLANZAPINE AND FLUOXETINE (SYMBYAX)

This drug is a combination of the atypical antipsychotic olanzapine and the selective serotonin reuptake inhibitor (SSRI) fluoxetine and is used to treat the depressive cycle of bipolar disease when other drugs have not been effective. It is usually taken once a day, with or without food. Fluoxetine can stay in the body for up to 5 weeks after the last dose. While treating depression can help prevent suicidal thoughts, some patients, usually those under age 25, will experience worsening depression or other mental symptoms (including mania) when taking this drug. This may worsen suicidal thinking and raise the risk of suicide, so any worsening of symptoms should be immediately reported. As with all SSRIs, it may take several weeks to see the full benefit of the antidepressant activity. Additional drug interactions due to the fluoxetine are present, in addition to the usual atypical antipsychotic interactions. One example is methylene blue, which increases seratonin levels and may produce toxicity. Any drug that increases seratonin levels or is an MAO inhibitor is contraindicated. The usual QT interval prolonging drug cautions exist. There is the potential for prolonged bleeding times in those taking aspirin, NSAIDs, or blood-thinning, antiplatelet drugs.

Side effects include dizziness, sleepiness, diarrhea, dry mouth, constipation, increased appetite, weight gain, elevated blood sugar/diabetes, and insomnia. Serious side effects include fainting, severe mental or mood changes, including suicidal thoughts, swelling of the extremities, tremor, extrapyramidal symptoms, a slow or irregular heartbeat, or signs of infection. Severe headache, seizures, neuroleptic malignant syndrome, priapism, and allergic reaction may also occur. Prolactin levels are increased in 28–47 percent of people taking this drug. SSRI side effects include decreased libido, lack of orgasm, erectile dysfunction, and abnormal ejaculation.

1st Generation (Typical) Antipsychotics

HALOPERIDOL (HALDOL, HALDOL DECANOATE, HALOPERIDOL LA, PERIDOL)

This drug is used on an acute basis to treat agitation in acute mania or psychosis and when given either IM or IV it begins to take effect within 30–60 minutes. When it is taken orally, peak blood levels occur in 2–6 hours and the half life of the drug is 10–20 hours. The long-acting intramuscular decanoate form of the drug peaks in 6–7 days, lasts 2–4 weeks, and has a half life of 3 weeks. The drug is metabolized in the liver and is excreted in the urine and feces. There is a risk of QT interval prolongation, and the usual drug cautions exist that are listed under the quetiapine (Seroquel) drug information. Since Haldol is sedating, additional sedating drugs will magnify this effect, including narcotics, belladonna, chloral hydrate, the benzodiazepenes, alcohol, ketamine, lithium, melatonin, barbiturates, propofol, henbane, skullcap, shepherd's purse, motherwort, and marijuana. Akathisia occurs in 60 percent and sedation, weight gain, and anticholinergic symptoms commonly occur. Extrapyramidal symptoms such as stiff muscles, Parkinsonian symptoms, and tardive dyskinesia may occur. Neuroleptic maligant syndrome is an infrequent complication, as are acute glaucoma, bone marrow suppression, severe hypotension, and allergic reaction.

LOXAPINE INHALED (ADASUVE)

This drug is used to treat acute agitation. It is inhaled once in a 24 hour period but there is a risk of bronchospasm so its use is restricted and it must be closely monitored and given only in the healthcare setting. Patients with pulmonary disease (asthma, COPD, etc.) should be screened for wheezing prior to administering this drug. COPD (chronic obstructive pulmonary disease) patients have a 19 percent risk of adverse effects, with 14 percent experiencing a distorted sense of taste. Sedation occurs in 12 percent, throat irritation in 3 percent, and bronchospasm, which can be severe enough to lead to respiratory arrest, in 0.8 percent. There is a small risk of akathisia and neuroleptic malignant syndrome. This drug lowers seizure threshold, may exacerbate glaucoma, and can trigger urinary retention.

Benzodiazepenes

These drugs treat anxiety and have a sedative effect, so they are used to treat acute mania or to abort emerging manic attacks. The most common side effects are cough, runny nose, muscle aches and pains, and various GI complaints such as diarrhea or constipation, and nausea, dyspepsia, or anorexia.

Hypotension can occur along with a rapid heart rate. A prolonged QTc interval, neuroleptic malignant syndrome, and increased prolactin levels may also occur. Examples of this drug category include Klonopin (clonazepam), Valium (diazepam), Xanax (alprazolam), Ativan (lorazepam), Librium (chlordiazepoxide), Tranxene (clorazepate), Dalmane (flurazepam), Doral (quazepam), Restoril (temazepam), Halcion (triazolam) and Serax (oxazepam).

Lorazepam is absorbed rapidly, peaks in 1 to 2 hours, and has a half life of 10 to 20 hours, so it is useful for treating acute anxiety. Clonazepam is absorbed slowly, peaks later, and has a half life of 18–50 hours, so it is more useful in treating chronic anxiety. Temazepam (Restoril), along with the nonbenzodiazepene drugs of zaleplon (Sonata) and zolpidem (Ambien), are used to treat insomnia, which can occur in both mania and depression. While benzodiazepenes are safer than other sedatives, like barbiturates, they can cause respiratory depression, which can be fatal when combined with narcotics or other sedating medications. Physical dependence and addiction can occur, and when an individual has been on these drugs for a long period of time, gradual weaning is necessary to prevent withdrawal. These drugs should be used with caution in anyone with a substance abuse problem, especially a problem with opiates like OxyContin (oxycodone), methadone, or heroin.

Anxiolytics

Any drug used to treat anxiety can be placed in this category, including the benzodiazepines, the antidepressants, and Buspar (buspirone), which is effective in treating generalized anxiety disorder by binding to specific serotonin receptors in the brain, as well as Vistaril (hydroxyzine), an antihistamine that is fast acting and reduces anxiety on an acute basis.

Antidepressants

Antidepressants are some of the most widely prescribed drugs in the United States, but their use in the treatment of bipolar depression is controversial because some antidepressants trigger a switch from depression to a manic or mixed mood state. Tricyclic antidepressants and monoamine oxidase inhibitors are more likely to cause a switch than the SSRIs, but all three categories of antidepressants are capable of switching. If a depressed person is treated with an antidepressant and begins to feel agitated and irritable, has trouble sleeping, or develops racing thoughts, this heralds the beginning of the switch to a mixed or manic mood state. When this happens, the antidepressant should be stopped and a different medication (a mood stabilizer) should be started in light of the new information that this individual has bipolar depression. There may be times when an antidepressant is needed for severe or unresponsive depression. In those situations, a mood stabilizer is nearly always given in conjunction with the antidepressant to protect against a manic switch. It can take up to 6 weeks for an antidepressant to work and close monitoring of every person placed on an antidepressant is vital, to watch for switching and for suicidal thinking, until the medication begins to take effect.

SSRIs

The SSRIs work by causing an increase in the neurotransmitter serotonin. The first was Prozac (fluoxetine), which I heard one person call his "happy pill" (he was clearly a bit hypomanic), followed by Zoloft (sertraline), Celexa (citalopram), Lexapro (escitalopram), and Paxil (paroxetine). Why are these drugs more popular then the old antidepressants? They have fewer side effects and are safer in general, so doctors feel more comfortable prescribing them because they don't worry as much about patients overdosing on them. The major complaint, however, is sexual dysfunction, vivid and intense dreams, and some irritability. Because these drugs affect the liver, they can affect other drugs that are broken down in the liver, like blood thinners, seizure medications, and blood pressure pills, so blood levels of these other drugs must be monitored.

SNRIs

SNRIs increase the amounts of the neurotransmitters serotonin and norepinephrine. Examples of this antidepressant category include Effexor and Effexor XR (venlafaxine), nefazodone (formerly Serzone, but the name brand as been withdrawn from the market), and Cymbalta (duloxetine).

TRICYCLICS

The tricyclic antidepressants also involve serotonin and norepinephrine and were the first antidepressants on the market but are rarely used today. Since they slow the electrical conduction of the heart, they are lethal if taken in overdose, causing cardiac arrest. They cause a number of side effects and may trigger mania or mixed episodes in a bipolar. They are mostly used today for unresponsive depression. Examples of this category of antidepressant are Elavil (amitriptyline), Ascendin (amoxapine), Anafranil (clomipramine), Norpramine (desipramine), Sinequan (doxepin), Tofranil (imipramine), Ludiomil (maprotiline), Pamelor (nortriptyline), and Vivactil (protriptyline).

MAOIs

The monoamine oxidase inhibitors affect the neurotransmitters epinephrine, norepinephrine, and dopamine. These drugs are rarely prescribed because of their side effects and dietary restrictions. In particular, foods containing tyramine may trigger a hypertensive crisis, therefore a long list of foods must be avoided, including aged cheeses like cheddar, red wine and ale, avocados if overripe, pineapples, eggplant, snow peas, aged, smoked, or marinated meats or fish, most pork (except for cured ham), processed meats, protein extracts, chocolate if eaten in excessive amounts, sour cream, yogurt, coconut, Brazil nuts, peanuts, yeast, and soy sauce. This drug can also trigger a switch from depression to a manic or mixed state. Examples of MAOIs are Nardil (phenelzine), Parnate (tranylcypromine), and Eldepryl or Emsam (selegiline).

Summary

1. It sometimes, but not always, takes a number of drugs to control bipolar disease.
2. The risks of untreated bipolar disease must be considered when contemplating the risks and benefits of bipolar medication.
3. There will almost always be side effects to deal with, but most are manageable.
4. Your bipolar medications will probably be changed from time to time, for a variety of reasons.
5. The goal of maintenance therapy is to maintain mood stabilization.
6. The antipsychotics treat acute mania or psychotic depression.
7. The atypical antipsychotics are sometimes used in maintenance therapy.
8. Benzodiazepenes are used for sedation, to acutely treat mania, or to treat anxiety or insomnia.
9. Antidepressants have a place in the treatment of bipolar for severe, unresponsive depression.
10. Always be honest with your mental health professional about your symptoms as well as your medication side effects.

Chapter 10

Talk Therapy and Lifestyle Management

Once your bipolar disease is consistently and effectively medicated, you are ready for the next two important steps of treatment. Each treatment step is important in the control of bipolar disease, and individuals who faithfully take their medication, participate in some form of talk therapy, and manage their lifestyle have the best chance of getting their bipolar into remission. You may be able to get by without one or perhaps two of the three main forms of treatment, but you won't be able to fully maximize your chances for recovery without all three; and you could be risking bipolar disaster if you cut corners in your treatment.

Talk Therapy (Psychotherapy)

This is one of the three important steps in bipolar treatment, in addition to medication and living a stable, regulated lifestyle. Although bipolar disease is biological in nature, the emotional symptoms and the behavior that results from these symptoms wreak havoc with the bipolar's personal and professional life. While treatment of the biological aspect of this disease is necessary, attention to the psychological ramifications of the disease is just as important if the bipolar is going to live a well balanced, fulfilled life with healthy, satisfying relationships. Studies have shown that bipolars who receive some form of talk therapy do better than those who don't; they are more likely to stay on their medications or notify their mental health professional when early symptoms develop. The end result is that they tend to get well faster and stay well longer.

Nearly all bipolars will benefit from some form of talk therapy, even if it's just a support group. One form of therapy appears to be as effective as another and a bipolar's needs may change as the illness changes over time, so their choice of talk therapy may also change over time (Schottle, Huber, and Bock). While all forms of talk therapy include psychoeducation, each type focuses on a specific aspect of bipolar functioning that may or may not apply to every bipolar, depending on whether they are recovering from a mood attack, are stable, are newly diagnosed, whether they have difficulties in their thinking or have behavioral problems, or suffer significant problems in their relationships at home or at work. Your mental health professional will guide you to the talk therapy that will best meet your specific needs at any given time during the course of your illness. Some therapists will use a combination of methods to address specific needs or use different therapies at different times when those needs change, while others specialize in only one type of therapy. The details don't matter as much as getting some form of therapy and committing to it. Don't be fooled, though. This isn't going to be a "lie on the couch and talk while the therapist takes notes" situation, although you may need that type of counseling at some point during your illness. You will learn, you will work, and you will change, always with the goal in mind of getting control over your disease. Results, if you commit to your therapy, can be incredible, life changing, and even life saving.

There are many ways a bipolar can benefit from talk therapy but one of the most important, at least in the beginning, is education. You cannot control a disease unless you know as much about that disease as you can. Not only do you need to know about bipolar disease in general, you also need to know how bipolar disease manifests in you in particular. Because the specific signs of an impending mood switch will be different for everyone, you will learn how to recognize your early symptoms of depression or hypomania and then you will learn what you can do to intervene before your mood gets out of control. You will learn about your medications so you will understand why and how they are important in the control of your disease. And because it is always difficult to adjust to the idea of living with a chronic illness requiring lifelong medication and lifestyle changes, you will have ample opportunity to talk about your feelings and to get the help and support you need in order to move forward with your recovery.

You will need a great deal of help regarding lifestyle management, including coping strategies to handle stress, particularly if you were self-medicating with alcohol or drugs or were relying on other abnormal coping mechanisms before you were diagnosed. You may need help in improving family, friend, or work relationships or to deal with guilt over some of the things you have done during bipolar attacks. If you don't have a strong support system at home, a therapist or support group can give you the support you need as you struggle to get a handle on your disease. You may have worries about passing the bipolar genes to your children, or how your illness will impact the future of your family or your ability to earn a living. And, finally, you may need help planning your future, once you know the vulnerabilities and strengths of your particular brand of bipolar. This disease is a lot to handle on your own and it makes sense that it might require several approaches in order to master it. There is no shame in getting as much help as you need, as often as you need it. Anything you can do to increase your chances for success should be embraced.

Different types of talk therapy will be discussed below and you will see the differences in approaches to similar problems. Some may appeal to you and others may not. Some types of therapy may be available in your community while others aren't. If you live in a city or large metropolitan area you will have many choices, but if you live in a small community you may have little choice in the talk therapy available to you. The type of therapy you choose isn't as important as the fact that you participate in some form of talk therapy. Even attending a support group is helpful, if no other options are available.

Cognitive Behavioral Therapy (CBT)

Cognitive behavioral therapy was originally designed for depression but was later adapted for other conditions, including bipolar disease, and is the most extensively tested and practiced form of talk therapy in use today. It is based on the concept that you can alter your moods by changing the way you think about your behavior. Instead of looking deep into the subconscious, conscious thought and attitudes are examined to see how they affect behavior, feelings, and moods. We've all heard the "put a smile on your face when you're feeling blue" axiom and this therapy is an example of that mindset.

I've spent a good deal of time in this book explaining to you that your moods are biologically based and not easily controlled by your thoughts and actions. Why, then, does this therapy help some bipolars, especially those who are depressed? The adaptation of this technique for bipolar disease assumes that stressful life events trigger negative habits of thought or action that either precipitate a mood switch or worsen one that is already occurring. In other words, you might not be able to completely control whether or not you have a depressive or hypomanic or manic mood swing, but you can change how you interpret things that happen in your life that might trigger or worsen those mood changes. Therefore you can change your behavior in an attempt to keep a mood swing mild or lessen its impact on your life. If you have heart disease and notice early signs of heart failure, you wouldn't think you were a hopeless case, destined to die of heart failure, would you? Instead you would take immediate action and call your doctor, expecting an adjustment in your heart medication would be prescribed to help alleviate your symptoms. CBT teaches you to look at your moods as a physical symptom of your disease so when you notice early symptoms, which will be different and specific for each bipolar, you will act on them before they worsen or before a crisis occurs.

For example, as soon as you feel the first stirrings of depression, you are likely to engage in negative thinking that may result in self-defeating behaviors that worsen your mood state. An example of distorted, negative thinking that often occurs in depression is that you are worthless, your environment or life is overwhelming, and nothing is ever going to change. CBT teaches you to stop this habit of negative thinking so you can attempt to intervene in your mood state. Instead of feeling hopeless, worthless, and victimized early in a depression, you might increase your exercise schedule, start light therapy, or contact your doctor for an adjustment in your medications. You can reduce your activities or workload so you won't feel overwhelmed, increase the activities that normally bring you pleasure, and avoid self-defeating behaviors you may have done in the past when you felt hopeless and depressed, like staying in bed during the day, overeating, or watching too much TV. By taking positive rather than negative action, you may be able to intervene early enough to keep your depression from worsening. In other words, you may not be able to change the way you feel but you may be able to change how you behave. Instead of over-identifying with your mood, you remain objective, identify what might have triggered your mood, and then make adjustments to your environment or schedule as necessary. Instead of feeling helpless and hopeless, you react in a proactive rather then a reactive way.

CBT can be helpful in the very early stages of hypomania by teaching the bipolar to do a reality check on their rising delusions of grandeur or lack of inhibitions. Because insight usually remains relatively intact in mild to moderate depression, CBT works better in depression than it does in hypomania and mania, which often come on so quickly that insight is lost before the bipolar recognizes what is happening. It is often very difficult for CBT to work in hypomania because the bipolar has to recognize what is going on in order to behave in a different way. They will have to be astute to notice when their thoughts are faster than usual or when they have the urge to spend more money than they normally do or when they have an unusual burst of energy. The hypomanic mood state is so enjoyable that the bipolar doesn't want it to stop, and these early signs often go unrecognized or ignored. That's why it's best to prevent the hypomanic state from occurring than to intervene after it has occurred.

CBT training will help you think about possible triggers if you begin to feel hypomanic. You may remember that you didn't get enough sleep the night before or you will recognize that you are under more stress than usual or perhaps you are overstimulated by your surroundings. You can make choices to keep your stimulation as low as possible, you can get to bed on time so that you get plenty of sleep until your symptoms improve, and you can choose to be extra careful about staying on schedule and taking your medications on time. Special coping mechanisms, like yoga or meditation, can be started or increased to help you handle stress, and you can decrease your daily activities until your mood normalizes. A spouse or trusted friend can handle your credit cards in order to limit spending until your hypomania has resolved. Instead of simply reacting to your hypomania without thinking, you can be proactive in handling your mood state.

Stephen Fry, in his documentary *The Secret Life of the Manic Depressive*, worried about his excessive shopping when he was manic, so he challenged a CBT therapist to keep him from buying things he didn't need. No matter what she said in an attempt to help him limit his spending, he always had an excuse for why he needed or wanted or deserved what he bought, even if he had multiple items of the same thing at home. He insisted he worked hard and he deserved whatever he was buying. He admitted to owning 9 digital cameras, although he had never used them, and he also owned 14–20 iPods (he couldn't remember the exact number), 5 video game systems, 12 computers, and, in the past, 11 motorcars. Fry purchased his 13th computer while the therapist asked him if he really needed yet another one, and at the end of this shopping spree with the therapist in tow, he gleefully boasted that he had "won" and the therapist had "lost" (*Stephen Fry: The Secret Life, Part 2*).

While Fry is luckier than most bipolars in that he is wealthy and can afford his manic shopping sprees, this isn't a game for most bipolars, whose excessive spending often puts them in serious financial peril. He was not a patient of this therapist nor had he gone through any real cognitive behavioral therapy; he had asked only for a demonstration of the techniques used to control hypomanic spending. The goal of therapy is to have the bipolar learn to think in the ways the therapist demonstrated for Fry so they can control their spending on their own. The therapist is neither a babysitter nor a policeman, there to play control games with the bipolar, but to help the bipolar learn to control mood-related behaviors independently.

CBT also teaches you to reward yourself for behaviors that may be difficult for you to do, but must be done in order to keep your disease under control. Important habits like taking your medication or going to bed on time may respond to behavior modification therapy techniques. CBT can also be very useful in helping set up a regular daily schedule you will actually follow. CBT is useful in treating anxiety and obsessive-compulsive disorder as well as depression, and it can help you handle stressors in a healthier way than you may be used to doing. For example, if you have an irrational fear about something, gradually increased exposure to what you are afraid of may help desensitize you (Miklowitz 129).

Dialectical Behavioral Therapy (DBT)

This form of therapy is similar to CBT but it involves emotions and interpersonal relationships, preventing the emotional arousal and overreaction that ruin so many interactions between bipolars and their friends, families, and coworkers. While this therapy was originally designed for those with borderline personality disorder, its usefulness in bipolar disease was soon recognized. The participant works with a therapist and then goes to a group session to practice interacting with others. Friends and family are allowed to participate in these group sessions if they so desire (Kahl, Winter, and Schweiger).

Interpersonal and Social Rhythm Therapy (IPSRT)

This therapy, which is sometimes combined with family focused therapy, was originally developed for depression but was modified for other disorders, including bipolar disease, as it focuses on social interaction and interpersonal relationships. The goal is not to alter the bipolar's personality but to address the social problems in the bipolar's life at the moment; past relationship issues are not dealt with and only current relationships are of interest. The behavioral aspect of a bipolar's dysfunctional social interactions or relationships are examined, and four main areas of social or interpersonal problem areas are considered potential triggers for mood episodes. The first is grief, which may be due to the death of a loved one, the loss of a special relationship or the loss of a sense of identity after diagnosis and medication. The second is interpersonal tension or separation, which may be caused by angry manic outbursts or other impulsive, disruptive manic behaviors. The third is role transition, which may be caused by a new job, relocating to a new house or a new school, the death of a spouse, a divorce, the birth of a baby, or any major life disruption. The fourth and last area is role deficiency, where the consequences of a manic or possibly a severe depressed episode or a suicide attempt causes a change in the way the bipolar is treated by friends, family, and coworkers (Frank).

Family Focused Therapy (FFT)/Couple's Therapy

Living with a bipolar can be difficult and the special needs a bipolar brings to the family dynamic can be disruptive and difficult for many families to handle. As I've said a number of times in this book, bipolar disease is a family disease, not only because it's inherited and other family members will likely be on the spectrum, but also because the bipolar's behavior can be excessive and at times so extreme the family is often kept in an uproar. This may be hard for many bipolars to comprehend, as they often don't view they behavior in the same way their families do. They often see themselves as exciting or passionate or stimulating as compared to their dull, average family. Families with a lot of emotion benefit greatly from this type of therapy, because bipolars who live in such families have a high relapse rate. The overinvolvement of the family with the bipolar, or perhaps the hostility or outright rejection aimed toward the bipolar, increases stress not only for the bipolar but also for the rest of the family.

This form of therapy includes those family members who are living with or dealing with the bipolar on a routine basis. Clearly, this is appropriate only if the bipolar has an interested, supportive family that is eager to learn about bipolar disease and wants to be involved in the bipolar's life. This therapy educates, helps with coping techniques as well as communication, and can help with problem solving within the family. Expressing both positive and negative emotions in a nonjudgmental way, learning active listening skills, and finding ways to ask for change are some of the communication skills taught in this form of therapy. The family also learns the importance of providing a calm, low-stress, nonstimulating home environment for the bipolar (Miklowitz 130–31).

Counseling

This is the traditional idea of therapy, where the patient talks and the counselor listens and is supportive although education and advice are offered as needed. Sometimes a bipolar simply needs to accept the reality of the disease or the fact that he will have to take medication for life. Other times there may be a great deal of guilt over past behavior, betrayals, mistakes, or hurts. Since bipolar is a family disease, the bipolar may have been raised by a bipolar parent and the childhood home might have been unstable. Sometimes physical or sexual abuse has occurred or other traumatic events have happened in the bipolar's life that are a source of stress and instability. Intensive therapy or counseling may be needed to resolve these issues before the bipolar can move forward, because deep issues have a way of eventually working to the surface if they are suppressed.

There are different types of counselors, with different educational experiences, from social workers with counseling training to psychologists as well as licensed professional counselors, marriage and family counselors, nurses with advanced degrees, DOs, PhDs, and MDs. So choose whomever you feel most comfortable with. You will know when you feel a connection with the person you are seeing. You can't build trust if you don't feel listened to and understood, and you can't fully trust someone you don't like. You have the right to "fire" a counselor, or any therapist, if you feel a trusting and supportive relationship isn't developing.

Group Therapy/Support Groups

Not everyone is comfortable sharing private information in a group setting, but many people feel a great deal of camaraderie when they share the same disease as others. They can "compare notes," problem solve, share information and resources, and sometimes just complain together. While it may be distressing to see others in the group worsen during an attack, it is also helpful to see them recover, and strategies for recovery and wellness can be shared within the group as well. For bipolars who lack close relationships with friends or family, these groups may be especially important as a source of understanding, validation, and support. Even bipolars with understanding friends and family find support groups to be incredibly helpful and a source of optimism and hope. There is a nationwide group called the Depression and Bipolar Support Alliance that sponsors support groups all over the country. You can learn if one is in your area by going to their website, which is listed in the resource section at the end of this book. Otherwise, call your local mental health provider or ask your mental health professional if there are support groups available in your area.

Recovery Wellness Plans

This form of therapy emphasizes the individual person rather than the mental health "system," where the bipolar might be seen merely as a diagnosis and not as an individual. In giving power back to the bipolar, individualization of treatment, recovery, and maintenance is maximized. Bipolars work with their strengths, called wellness tools, rather than their weaknesses, and look to other recovered bipolars for help and support. These programs are supported by research and are evidence-based practices. Two types of Recovery Wellness programs are discussed below.

Illness Management and Recovery Program (IMR)

This program is free of charge and is available from the Substance Abuse and Mental Health Administration (SAMHSA), a government organization.

The mentally ill are taught how to make their needs known and how to choose their doctor or therapist based on their specific needs. Self-directed wellness plans are encouraged, along with crisis plans in case of a mental health emergency. Each treatment plan is therefore highly specific and individualized. Mistakes are expected, acknowledged, and used as learning experiences (Mueser, Corrigan, and Hilton).

Wellness Recovery Action Plan (WRAP)

Participants in this recovery plan use wellness tools that play to their strengths to ward off mood escalation when symptoms develop. A crisis plan is developed so family members know what the participant wants them to do if that person is no longer able to make her own decisions. A post-crisis plan is also in place so a return to a state of wellness can proceed according to the participant's wishes. The focus is on education, hope, personal responsibility, self-advocacy, and support, with the goal of mental health, quality of life, and adequate social functioning, in addition to treatment and recovery, when mood attacks occur. WRAP groups vary in size but generally contain from 8 to 12 members, with two trained leaders who demonstrate the WRAP concept in their own lives. There are normally 8 weekly sessions that last 2 hours each, but this may vary and groups that bond may continue to meet after the official 8-week training is over. Materials for the course are relatively inexpensive but leader training is costly ("Wellness Recovery"; Copeland).

Assertive Community Treatment Teams (ACTTs)

These teams are often provided by the local community mental health provider for those who are severely or chronically mentally ill. While not all areas have an ACTT, and not all ACTTs provide all of the services listed below, you can call your local community mental health provider to learn if ACTT is available in your area and if so, what services are provided. Some ACTTs accept self-referrals but others require referral by a physician or mental health professional. These teams are made up of different specialists who can provide a variety of services in order to keep individuals out of the hospital and living as normal a life as possible. The range of services provided not only covers psychiatric care, but may also include finding a home for those who are homeless, acquiring medication when there is an inability to pay or a lack of insurance, supervising medication, and finding suitable employment for those without a job. Contact with the ACTT can be daily or sometimes as often as several times a day if medication supervision is required. Help with insurance or vocational and educational rehabilitation is sometimes offered. There is usually a 24-hour crisis hot-line available ("ACT Model").

Lifestyle Management

This is the third and final necessary bipolar treatment option. First, you need medication, and you need it every day. Second, you need some form of talk therapy. You may need a little or you may need a lot, a few lucky individuals may not need much at all. Nearly everyone most certainly needs some, especially early on, when they are first trying to get their disease under control. Talk therapy will educate you about the disease and help you begin to make lifestyle changes. But medication and talk therapy aren't going to work as well as they could unless you get your daily schedule under control. I know this goes against the essence of your bipolar personality but that's the very reason you must try so hard to get a firm grip on this aspect of your life.

Andy Behrman's bipolar spiraled out of control, seemingly unresponsive to medication. When he realized he had become addicted to electroconvulsive therapy (ECT), or at least to the sedative and anesthesia given prior to his treatments, he realized he had to stop ECT. Behrman, like many bipolars, had neglected to make significant lifestyle changes in order to tame his out-of-control disease. Once Behrman was out of treatment options, he had no choice but to submit to his mental health professional's advice about making significant changes in how he lived his life. With expert guidance, counseling, and education, what had seemed like a hopeless case of bipolar was tamed by the treatment option Behrman had discounted as being unimportant and not worthy of his effort and attention. The medications that he thought were ineffective worked perfectly once he began to live a stable, regulated life. When Behrman committed to changing his lifestyle, the results were no less than miraculous.

You inherited genes that made you susceptible to having bipolar disease. These genes set you up for a lack of regulation in your brain that result in your moods swinging from one extreme to the other. Your bipolar medications work in various ways to regulate these moods because your brain is unable to do so without help. While it is easy to describe bipolar disease as a chemical imbalance, your inherited biological dysregulation is much more complicated than just abnormal levels of neurotransmitters. There are problems with information processing between nerve cells and between different areas of the brain as well as problems with the biological clock that regulates your sleep-wake cycle and other body functions. Because bipolar disease is a biological dysregulation brain disease, environmental triggers such as stress, drug or alcohol use, too much or too little sunlight, erratic use of your bipolar medication, or too little or too much sleep can trigger mood episodes. The more serious mood triggers will be discussed below as well as some of the lifestyle management strategies that are necessary to get your bipolar disease under control.

Life Stressors

Moodiness may be an inherent part of your personality and this moodiness may sometimes expand into mood states that may seem to come and go for no obvious reason. But "life stressors" can also occur that take advantage of your underlying brain dysregulation, so that even your bipolar medications may not be able to prevent a mood episode, although hopefully they will help keep the episodes from getting out of control. Bipolar individuals vary in susceptibility to these life stressors. Some will remain relatively stable and are threatened only by major stressors like divorce or the death of a spouse or the loss of a job, while others may be threatened by less severe stressors like having a difficult day at work, harsh words with a friend, or getting stuck in traffic. Life stressors are difficult and may cause mood changes in everyone, not just the bipolar. Because of the biological, inherited problem with mood regulation that bipolars must struggle with on a daily basis, bipolars are more sensitive to life stressors, both large and small, than those without bipolar disease and are more likely to have extreme moods as a result of those stressors.

During a period of remission when the mood state is stable, bipolars may be relatively resilient to some life stressors, depending on their underlying sensitivity and the severity of the stressor, but as stressors accumulate, symptoms of a mood switch may begin to emerge. Some bipolars may be able to live a relatively normal life, handling minor changes in their daily routine or minor stressors without triggering symptoms, while others may need a strict daily schedule and as little stress as possible in order to keep their symptoms under control. But even the most resilient of bipolars can be thrown by a major life stressor. No matter how hard anyone tries, bipolar or not, none of us can control what life may throw at us. We all need coping strategies when major life stressors invade our lives or when stress builds up, but bipolars need coping skills on a daily basis because of their inherent susceptibility to mood destabilization.

For the bipolar, even a positive life event may serve as a life stressor in that getting overly excited may trigger hypomania or mania. Happy events like a job promotion, a new romantic relationship, or inheriting money activates the reward area of the brain. A non-bipolar person feels elated for a time at their good fortune but eventually calms down. A bipolar becomes elated and then dysregulated because their brain isn't able to keep their elated mood in check. Their mood may continue to rise until it reaches hypomanic or manic levels. Conversely, a negative life change, like the death of a loved one or the loss of a job, may trigger abnormal dopamine and seratonin activity in the brain, causing depression. While a non-bipolar person may also feel depressed under these circumstances, the depression usually won't deepen as much as the depression of a bipolar, and it definitely won't switch into hypomania, mania, or a mixed state once the depression has lifted.

Life stressors, both large and small, must be watched for and dealt with daily. Likewise, early symptoms of a mood episode must be constantly monitored and, when detected, must be dealt with appropriately. For example, if stressors begin to accumulate, meditation and yoga can be incorporated into the daily schedule or increased if they are already a part of the schedule. Work or social obligations may be decreased until the stress has resolved. If early signs of depression are noted, aerobic activity can be started or increased. If hypomania threatens, the noise level in the house can be kept down. Family members can be instructed that shouting, stomping around, door banging, or loud music and TV is forbidden until the bipolar is feeling better. When stressors begin to accumulate and mood symptoms emerge, the daily schedule needs to tighten up and stay relatively rigid until these symptoms resolve and the life stressors are gone. Going to bed on time and getting up on time becomes even more important than usual when trying to avoid a mood episode. At least 8 hours of sleep a night is needed; but sleeping too much, as often happens during depression, cannot be allowed to occur. Mealtimes should be regular and, of course, the medication schedule should be like clockwork.

It seems that many bipolars are drawn to professions, people, and lifestyles that are filled with chaos and noise and energy and creativity and stimulation. Just as many bipolars identify with their manic personalities, they also identify with their manic lifestyles. When depressed or when relatively stable and neither up or down, they will often have difficulty keeping up with their manic lifestyle or their wild and noisy friends. The things or people they sought out and found so stimulating and fun while hypomanic or manic suddenly become overstimulating and stressful when they are in a mixed, depressed or neutral state. Marya Hornbacher said this about her very manic writer's lifestyle, as she began to sink into a depression and couldn't keep up with the pace of her life anymore: "[M]y life is chaotic. If there was no chaos in my life, there'd be no chaos in my head" (106). Although she had been diagnosed with bipolar disease some years earlier and took her meds from time to time, usually when feeling depressed, she thought her hypomanic personality was her real identity, and that her chaotic, hard-drinking lifestyle was a typical writer's way of living because her eccentric and erratic behavior was tolerated due to her brilliance as a writer. She sought help only when she couldn't keep up with her manic lifestyle as her mood dropped.

Biological Clock Disruption

Triggering events or lifestyle changes can disrupt the biological clock, which resides in the anterior hypothalamus in the brain, and runs at slightly more than 24 hours, as compared to the 24-hour earth rotation on which we base our time clocks. This internal biological clock coordinates with external signals from the environment, particularly light and dark via the retina in the back of our eyes, to affect a number of complex body processes, from wakefulness to internal body temperature to hormone production to blood pressure. This roughly 24-hour fluctuation of body functions, controlled by the biological clock, is called the circadian rhythm.

The pineal gland, located in the center of the brain, produces melatonin in the absence of mainly blue light (think blue skies) and suppresses production of this hormone in the presence of blue light. This light shines (or doesn't shine) on the retina in the back of the eyes, which signals the pineal gland to suppress (or produce) melatonin, which then signals the internal biological clock in the hypothalamus to cause the body changes connected to the circadian rhythm. Incandescent lights are yellow and if these lights are kept dim at night, they won't affect melatonin production. The blue light from TV, computer and smart phone screens could suppress melatonin production and disrupt the circadian rhythm. Dr. Sis has strong ideas about sleep and bipolar:

> I believe sleep is the key to being stable and highly functional. Every time I have decompensated and ended up locked in a hospital or a jail, I mean EVERY TIME, it has been because of insomnia. I do not sleep without medication. Since the 80's. I believe that sleep deprivation is the key to this whole disease. Go back to the neurotransmitters. Melatonin, seratonin ... sleep.

For a bipolar who most likely inherited a gene causing some type of malfunction of the biological clock, losing just a night or two of sleep may bring on hypomania. While you may not be able to prevent all of the triggers in your life, you can prevent this one by going to bed on time and getting up on time so you keep your hours of sleep the same every night. This also means keeping the same schedule on weekends as you do during the week. While others may skimp on sleep during the work week and sleep in on weekends, you won't be able to do that because catching up on sleep or sleeping more on weekends than you do during the week will upset your already sensitive biological clock. The same can be said for napping. If you nap each day as part of your daily routine and don't have any problem going to sleep at bedtime, then naps are fine for you. But if you don't normally nap and then decide to take a long nap one day, you risk getting off schedule if you can't fall asleep that night.

Sometimes getting to bed on time isn't the problem, rather, going to sleep or staying asleep is what's difficult. There are many tricks to help you ease into feeling restful and ready for sleep once you are nearing your bedtime. First of all, don't stress over whether you feel sleepy or not. Some people feel drowsy before they go to bed and fall asleep quickly while others feel wide awake and need to root around for 10, 15, or even 20 minutes in bed before they begin to fall asleep. Avoid excess stimulation before bedtime, and keep the lights low. You can read or watch TV as long as it doesn't stimulate you so much that it makes it harder for you to fall sleep. Even though experts caution about the blue light from your computer, smart phone, or TV suppressing melatonin, which means you won't feel sleepy at bedtime, there are many people who fall asleep in front of the TV, so use common sense to know what works best for you. Melatonin tablets are available over the counter to help you feel sleepy before bedtime, but they interfere with some bipolar medications. If you decide to try them, be sure to talk to your mental health professional first.

Stimulants such as caffeine or decongestants, or substances that interfere with sleep quality, like alcohol or spicy foods, should be avoided before bedtime. Some people are more sensitive to caffeine than others and having any caffeine after 5:00 or even 3:00 p.m. may prevent sleepiness at 10:00 or 11:00 p.m. A wind-down period of 1–2 hours before bedtime is recommended, preferably without TV or computer or smart phones, unless those activities put you to sleep. Reading a book makes some people sleepy unless the book is so exciting it keeps them awake. Be sure to turn off any alerts or sounds on your cell phone, computer, or tablet, because these noises could wake you at night or interfere with the quality of your sleep. Make sure your bedroom temperature is comfortable and the noise level is acceptable. Wear ear plugs or use a fan or white noise machine if there are noises that keep you awake. In some cases, a pill to help you sleep may be needed for the occasional sleepless night but this shouldn't become a routine practice unless it is the only way you can get to sleep. Your mental health professional should be the one to prescribe any sleeping medication you need.

What do you do if traveling takes you to another time zone? If you are going to be only an hour or two off your own time zone, you can stay on your own time and eat and exercise and get up and go to bed on your original time rather than the time zone where you are. For a large difference in time zones it is suggested that bipolars prepare by shifting their schedule ahead or behind, depending on what is required, until the schedule matches the time zone of where they will travel. Dark sunglasses should be worn during the night hours of the prospective travel time zone if it's still daylight where they are so the pineal gland won't suppress melatonin production, thus helping the biological clock to reset. Unfortunately, this usually works best prior to a trip when you have weeks to gradually reset your biological clock to the new time zone. There usually isn't enough time to readjust before you come home, if you are traveling for only a week or two or you don't have a lot of control over your schedule while traveling. If you are staying in the new time zone for an extended period of time and have control of your schedule, you can begin to readjust to your home time zone before traveling back home.

Your Daily Schedule

Establishing and then keeping a regular daily schedule will go a long way in controlling your daily moodiness as well as preventing mood episodes. In addition to regular activities that include exercise, meals, taking medication, and socializing, additional activities can be added as needed to help alter mood states as they arise. Many of the talk therapies mentioned earlier in this chapter will help you establish a regular and stable daily schedule. If you aren't participating in talk therapy at the moment, your mental health provider can assist you in this task. First, the therapist or mental health professional will become as familiar as possible with your previous attacks as well as your most recent one and will get to know your normal daily routine in order to see if a pattern exists that might be triggering episodes. It is extremely important for you to be as honest as you can with the person helping you. Your professional or therapist has heard it all before, so you shouldn't be embarrassed or worried about what they will think of you. If you routinely get only a few hours of sleep at night, drink too much or use drugs or take your medications sporadically, own up to it. The only way your therapist or professional can help you get better is to know what your current lifestyle is so they will know where you need to start to make changes. Don't worry—you won't be forced to move faster than you are willing or able to move.

Once a clear picture of your normal daily schedule has been established, a schedule will be set up that maximizes stability while retaining as much of your individual routine and personal lifestyle as possible. Your job is to gradually transition to this stable schedule in order to regulate your internal body clock. No one expects you to accomplish this overnight and your therapist or professional will help you make small but important changes until you have completely conquered your new schedule. Once that has been accomplished, anything that upsets this regular schedule will be dealt with. It may take several years to work out all the kinks in your new schedule since life can and often does throw curve balls. You will have plenty of support with the help of your therapist or professional so that one day you will know how to handle future curve balls by yourself. Eventually you will no longer need your therapist and will be capable of maintaining your regular schedule without help.

While it may seem like an easy thing to establish a stable schedule, following that schedule day in and day out is a difficult proposition. There are some people who are naturally scheduled people, who don't have to work at getting up at the same time every day, going to bed at the same time every night, eating meals on time, exercising or socializing or doing anything else on a schedule. While there may be rare exceptions to this rule, I would venture to say that these people are not bipolars. Without a properly functioning biological clock, there is no tendency or desire to follow a strict daily schedule. Doing so may be one of the hardest things you will have to do, perhaps even harder than taking your medications. This is why keeping a daily schedule is often one of the last things a bipolar is willing to do. As with any new habit, it takes time for any new routine to become as automatic as brushing your teeth or taking a shower—and I bet a lot of bipolars skip those things, too. Don't believe the old saying that it takes 6 weeks to develop a new habit. You get used to a habit in 6 weeks, but it's still awfully easy to drop a new habit at that point. Overhauling a daily schedule is more than just a new habit: it's a series of new habits and it may take a year or more for a new schedule to feel natural and normal.

In establishing a schedule, try to tag meals or bedtimes or taking medication or the time you wake up with something or someone in your household, at least in the beginning. If you live with someone who is very scheduled, you will have an easier time of it. They will likely have set times when they do their daily routine and you can follow them as they go about their day. If you live with people who aren't scheduled, then you are going to have a more difficult time setting your schedule. You can time your meals to certain TV shows, and if you work, the time you get up in the morning or go to bed at night will probably depend on your work schedule. If you are a student, try to set your class schedule the same every day, if possible. You will need to set up your exercise or social schedule to avoid excess stimulation near your bedtime. Shift work or erratic work hours should be avoided and your weekend hours need to be as similar to your weekday hours as possible. You may be able to relax your schedule a bit now and then, but in the beginning, until you get your bipolar under control, you need to start out as strictly as possible. There will always be life events, like a new baby, a new job, a new relationship, or travel to a different time zone, that will throw your schedule off. You will learn through experience how well you will be able to handle getting off schedule, but learning what you can do to stabilize yourself when you can't stay on schedule is an important way of learning how to take care of your bipolar disease.

Taking your medication every day is an important part of your daily schedule. Pills that are taken once or twice a day are easier to remember than ones you take three times a day. It's relatively easy to incorporate pill taking into a morning routine (assuming you get up at the same time each morning, as you should be doing), and the evening dose can be tied to some evening activity. Morning pills can be left by the sink and taken when you brush your teeth or at breakfast. Evening pills can be taken at dinner or as you sit down to watch TV after dinner. Midday pills are trickier, especially if you will be away from home. It's easy to get distracted and forget to take pills at lunch or, worse, at an odd time in the afternoon if no activity is linked to pill time. My family member sets the cell phone alarm to go off at pill time so a concrete reminder is always there, whether at home or away, and a few doses of medication are carried at all times so the medication is available when the alarm goes off.

Working Toward Remission

While I have given you ideas about some of the things that can be done to help manage your disease and listed some therapy options, you will have to choose what is right for you, based on what is available in your area, what you can afford, and what feels right for your situation. Each bipolar is different. Each of you will have different stressors, different underlying biological vulnerabilities, different ways that hypomania or depression begin to manifest, and different support systems. Within this broad framework, there are many individual paths to remission. But when it comes down to it, you are the one who is going to have to do the work. Your brain doesn't function as it should and there are things you can do to help it function better. But those things are going to require a daily, ongoing effort in order for you to succeed at getting control over your brain. Trust me: it's worth it.

Summary

1. Talk Therapy is an important aspect of bipolar treatment and there are many options available to suit each individual's need.
2. Cognitive Behavioral Therapy (CBT) suggests that you can change the way you behave during mood states to lessen the impact of that mood state on your life.
3. Dialectical Behavioral Therapy (DBT) and Interpersonal and Social Rhythm Therapy (IPSRT) focus on interpersonal relationships and social interactions.

4. Family Focused Therapy (FFT) and Couple's Therapy help provide a low-stress, calm, supportive home environment with good communication and problem solving.

5. Counseling is sometimes needed to work through issues of guilt, childhood trauma, physical or sexual abuse, or acceptance of having a chronic disease.

6. Group therapy or support groups can be valuable sources of support and camaraderie but can also provide education and problem solving.

7. Recovery Wellness Plans, such as the Illness Management and Recovery Plan (IMR) and the Wellness Recovery Action Plan (WRAP), teach advocacy and personal responsibility and are individualized to the bipolar's strengths.

8. Assertive Community Treatment Teams (ACTTs) offer a variety of services and are often provided by a community mental health provider for the chronically mentally ill.

9. Lifestyle management is an extremely important part of bipolar treatment and includes monitoring for and controlling life stressors, regulating the biological clock, and setting up a regular and stable daily schedule.

10. Achieving remission in bipolar disease requires medication, talk therapy, and lifestyle changes.

Chapter 11

Other Treatments

While medication, lifestyle changes, and talk therapy are the most important treatments an individual can pursue to gain control over bipolar disease, there are supplemental treatments or activities that may also help. Some are relatively minor and only assist the major therapies while others may play a more important role in the management of bipolar disease. None of the following supplemental treatments replaces the three major therapies discussed in the previous chapters and none should be undertaken without the knowledge of your mental health professional.

Dietary Changes, Vitamins, and Herbal Supplements

Regardless of whether one is healthy or suffering from any type of chronic disease, including a psychiatric illness, optimal nutrition is encouraged. While no particular diet has been found to specifically improve bipolar disease, a varied and healthy diet can improve the physical and mental health of nearly anyone. In general, what is good for the heart is also good for the brain, and eating regular, well balanced meals is as good for your mood and brain health as it is for your body. When you make simple, healthy dietary changes, you will likely be surprised at the improvement in your mood and energy level during the day. While dietary changes won't take away bipolar mood episodes, a positive change in your daily mood is a good start.

It is often said that our Western diet is healthy and nutritional deficiencies are rare because our food is plentiful, varied, and vitamin-enriched, yet most us don't eat a well balanced diet. Many of us skip at least one meal a day—usually breakfast—and while fresh, healthy food is available to most of us, it is often expensive and takes time to prepare. Too many of us do not ingest any sort of vegetable on a routine basis, or cook, so we resort to ready-made packaged foods or fast food eaten on the go. It's easier to get our meals through a drive-through than to go home and prepare a meal from scratch. And while reasonably healthy options are now available at most fast food or restaurant locations, we continue to choose the less healthy, traditional menu items.

We need a healthy diet in order to have the stamina, energy, and brain power to make it through our long and busy days. We grab candy bars and caffeine-loaded drinks to keep our energy levels up but the plummeting blood sugar and energy crash that follow force us to reach for yet more sugar and caffeine as we continue this repetitive cycle. We are often sleep deprived and chronically fatigued, and the roller coaster of our sugar levels and shifting wakefulness naturally affects our moods. We understand that we can treat our flagging energy levels or our sleepiness with food or drink; but we don't seem to realize that we can prevent this from happening, or at least minimize it, by feeding our bodies properly in the first place. Snacks of protein rather than sugar or caffeine keep the blood sugar stable and avoid the crash that brings on fatigue, sleepiness, irritability, and sugar cravings.

Other than general dietary advice, a few specific nutritional concerns involving some of the bipolar medications are listed below. Some nutrients affect the nervous system. While these are rarely deficient in our Western diet, in rare circumstances their levels may be decreased and cause symptoms. Although these low nutrient levels are more likely to involve neuropathy-like symptoms, depression or fatigue may also sometimes occur. Other nutrients are more closely related to moods or certain aspects of bipolar disease. Supplements should be taken with caution and discussed with your mental health professional, however, and none of these supplements replaces traditional bipolar therapy. Although you may consider herbal supplements natural and safe, some may interact with your bipolar medications and a few have the ability to induce mania. If they are effective enough to alter your mood state, even just a little, they should be considered drugs, even if they aren't as effective as your bipolar medications. When combined with other drugs you may be taking, unpleasant or dangerous side effects may occur.

Sodium/Salt Balance for Those on Lithium

Changes in salt (sodium chloride) intake must be avoided in individuals on lithium because fluctuating sodium levels may alter blood lithium levels, resulting in levels that are either too high, which can cause toxicity, or too low, which can mean the lithium won't work to control your bipolar disease. Prepackaged foods usually contain a great deal of sodium, so you must be careful to read labels so you will know how much sodium you will be consuming if you eat these types of food products. Restaurant or fast food meals contain variable amounts of salt, so you can't control the amount you are ingesting when you eat away from home. Cooking at home allows you better control over the amount of sodium in your food, and you can purchase reduced sodium products such as soups or soy sauce in order to control your daily sodium intake. You aren't aiming for a low sodium lifestyle—you simply need to keep your daily sodium levels relatively stable.

Elevated Blood Sugar and Blood Lipids for Those on Atypical Antipsychotics

The atypical antipsychotics sometimes cause metabolic syndrome, which is defined by either type 2 diabetes or an elevated fasting blood sugar level, elevated triglycerides, a reduced HDL cholesterol level, hypertension, and central obesity. Individuals who develop this problem will have to make dietary changes to control their lipids as well as their blood sugar. Eating healthy fats and complex carbohydrates and limiting simple starches and sugars not only keeps blood sugar under control but also helps improve the lipid profile. While not everyone on an atypical antipsychotic will develop this problem, appropriate dietary changes that are livable and acceptable can be started before strict dietary measures become mandatory. This may help delay or prevent metabolic syndrome from occurring in susceptible individuals.

Omega–3 Fatty Acids

Omega–3 fatty acids are not manufactured by the body and must be obtained solely from our diet. There are two types: eicosapentaenoic acid (EPA) and docosahexaenoic acid (DHA). High levels of these fatty acids are found in cold water fish such as salmon, mackerel, tuna, herring, sardines, and anchovies, but they are also in other foods such as walnuts and flaxseed oil, dark green leafy vegetables (spinach and arugula), and also game meats (deer and buffalo). Even free range chickens, eggs, and milk advertised with omega–3 enhancement contain some of these important fatty acids.

Some studies show that bipolar depression (but not mania) appears to be improved by omega–3 fatty acids (Sarris, Mischoulon, and Schweitzer), while other studies suggest these fatty acids help decrease the dosage of antipsychotic medications in individuals with psychosis. They also seem to delay or prevent the progression of psychosis in young people who have signs of early psychosis but who aren't fully psychotic yet (they hear voices or think someone is trying to read their mind). Perhaps these fatty acids are neuroprotective against oxidative stress, or maybe they alter cell membrane function (cell membranes are composed of fatty acids). There may also be some form of interaction with the neurotransmitters dopamine and serotonin. Whatever the mechanism, the researchers believed there is enough evidence to recommend a standard daily dose of fish oil be added to the medication regimen of all patients with psychosis (Amminger, Schäfer, and Papageorgiou).

Unless your diet contains a great deal of fish, you are unlikely to get enough of the omega–3 fatty acids to treat depression or psychosis, so supplementation is required. While this is a relatively safe supplement, it is still important to inform your mental health professional of your intent to use it, which should always be used in conjunction with your regular bipolar medication regimen, and at standard doses, as high doses may increase the risk of bleeding. Choose a supplement with a high purity rating and one without an unpleasant fishy aftertaste.

The B Vitamins

VITAMIN B1 (THIAMINE)

Our bodies are unable to produce Vitamin B1, or thiamine, and can only store a limited amount, mostly in the skeletal muscles, although it can also found in the brain, liver, kidneys, and heart. A wide variety of foods contain thiamine, but other foods, such as clams, mussels, fresh fish, shrimp, and milled rice, decrease absorption. Thiamine deficiency is rare in this country but can sometimes occur in chronic alcoholism, starvation, or gastric bypass surgery, and in those with absorption issues such as severe and prolonged diarrhea, severe vomiting, dialysis, chronic intestinal disease, and diuretic therapy, or through depletion of the body's thiamine stores because of high consumption that may occur in fever, pregnancy, physical exercise, carbohydrate or fat loaded diets, or hyperthyroidism.

As with all the B vitamins, thiamine is important for a healthy nervous system. If a deficiency of this vitamin is present, significant neurological problems can occur such as Beriberi, or Wernicke's encephalopathy or Korsakoff syndrome in the alcoholic. Treatment of deficiency usually requires several daily intramuscular injections of 50 mg thiamine until symptoms improve and then oral maintenance therapy at 2.5 to 5 mg per day unless there is an underlying condition that prevents the absorption of thiamine from the intestine. High energy states (hyperthyroidism, pregnancy) may require larger daily doses, but this supplement is generally safe, even at high doses, as long as renal function is good.

VITAMIN B6 (PYRIDOXINE)

A true deficiency of B6 is extremely rare, but decreased levels can sometimes be seen in the elderly, in alcoholism, and in severe malnutrition. The risk for pyridoxine deficiency is increased in inflammatory conditions such as rheumatoid arthritis and celiac disease, in those with previous intestinal surgery, in liver disease including hepatitis and liver cancer, in renal failure with dialysis or kidney transplant, or with certain medications. Psychiatric symptoms include depression and irritability. Since pyridoxine is abundant in a wide variety of foods, a well-balanced diet should provide most people with the recommended 2 mg daily intake. If an underlying physical problem is present that interferes with absorption, higher doses are needed, which can vary from 2.5 mg to 500 mg per day. Elevated levels of pyridoxine can cause a neuropathy that may result in searing foot pain and a staggering gait. While this complication is usually related to very high doses, it has occurred at doses of 50 mg a day, so a physician is required to determine the appropriate dose needed to correct a deficiency.

Vitamin B12 (Cobalamin)

There has been a long association between a lack of this vitamin and serious and sometimes irreversible brain, spinal cord, and peripheral nerve malfunction due to its involvement in neurotransmitter synthesis, the making and maintenance of myelin, and possibly a cytotoxic (cell-killing) mechanism. While the usual symptoms of B12 deficiency are numbness and tingling in the hands and feet, psychiatric and behavioral symptoms may occur in 8 percent of patients. These symptoms include hypomania, depression, psychosis with hallucinations and paranoia, emotional lability, and violence.

B12 deficiency is almost always caused by a lack of stomach intrinsic factor, which is needed for the body to absorb this vitamin from the diet. This is usually due to an autoimmune condition where antibodies attack gastric intrinsic factor. Inadequate dietary intake may also cause deficiency (fad diets, alcoholism), as does disease of the terminal ileum (Crohns, Celiac disease, surgery), lack of stomach acid (atrophic gastritis, reflux medication use), certain medications (colchicine, neomycin), or increased B12 requirement (hyperthyroidism, nitrous oxide exposure during anesthesia, or "whippet" abuse).

B12 is contained in meat, eggs, cheese and yogurt and if poor diet is to blame for deficiency, eating these foods rather than supplementation is the recommended course of action. If a condition preventing proper absorption is present, then parenteral doses (shots) may be required in order to completely avoid the intrinsic factor pathway. If no hindrance to small intestine absorption is present, a large oral dose will supply an adequate daily dose because a small amount (1 percent) will bypass the intrinsic factor pathway and be absorbed in the terminal ileum of the small intestine.

Folate (Folic Acid) Deficiency

Folate deficiency is rare because folate is found in many vegetables, fruits and animal products, as well as fortified packaged foods (such as cereal). However, malnutrition, chronic alcoholism, abnormal intestinal absorption, decreased metabolism (hypothyroidism, some drugs), increased metabolism requirement (pregnancy, hyperthyroidism), and increased excretion due to B12 deficiency may ultimately result in folate deficiency. Symptoms of deficiency include sleeplessness, irritability and forgetfulness. Neural tube defects in newborns have long been associated with this deficiency and there is also evidence for an increased risk of autism and diabetes-associated birth defects. Pre- and postnatal vitamins containing adequate levels of folate are prescribed for the pregnant and newly delivered mother in order to prevent these problems.

Folate supplementation in the older adult appears to reduce the risk of stroke but not cardiac events. Unfortunately, there is evidence that folate may increase the risk of developing cancer. Interestingly, the elderly, who are in the highest risk group for cancer, are the group most likely to over-supplement, and women of childbearing age and non–Hispanic black women, who most need adequate folate levels, are the groups most likely to under-supplement.

Vitamin D

Despite early excitement about a possible link between low levels of Vitamin D and depression, it has been proven that treating Vitamin D deficient depressed patients with high supplemental doses is no more effective than placebo treatment. This implies that Vitamin D deficiency may be caused by depression (perhaps the depressed stay indoors more than the non-depressed) rather than being the cause of depression.

5-HTP (5-Hydroxytryptophan)

This substance provides the building blocks for serotonin, so it may increase serotonin levels in the brain. It appears possibly to be effective for depression and fibromyalgia. There is a long list of drug interactions associated with 5-HTP, so don't take this supplement without your mental health professional's knowledge. Side effects are mostly GI-related, with loss of appetite, diarrhea, nausea, vomiting, heartburn, stomach pain, and gas.

Melatonin

This is a hormone produced in the pineal gland, which is an endocrine gland located near the center of the brain but outside the brain itself and therefore outside the blood brain barrier. This hormone is directly released into the systemic blood circulation and its release is triggered by darkness and inhibited by exposure to blue light. It is used for benzodiazepine or nicotine withdrawal, migraine and cluster headache prophylaxis, resetting the internal body clock when traveling through time zones, and treating jet lag or sleep-wake disorders, including those that occur with shift work. There is a long list of drugs that may interact with this hormone, including some bipolar drugs, so be sure you discuss this supplement with your mental health professional if you choose to use it. If taken at the wrong time or at too high a dose, excessive sleepiness, dizziness, daytime fatigue, or decreased alertness may occur.

St. John's Wort (Hypericum perforatum)

This herbal supplement may be effective in mild or moderate depression and has been used to treat obsessive-compulsive disorder and anxiety, but study results have been variable. While some have shown it to be more effective than placebo and even as effective as Prozac in treating depression, others have shown no advantage over placebo. This herb may cause mania in some bipolars, and it also interacts with some bipolar medications along with many other drugs. Due to the risk of mania, it is not recommended in bipolar disease or psychosis or for use in those with Alzheimer's disease. Allergic reactions may occur and this supplement may reduce the blood levels of oral contraceptives and other drugs. Side effects include skin rashes, headache, stomach upset, fatigue, and restlessness.

Valerian (Amantilla, All Heal)

This supplement is used to treat sleep disorders and insomnia, anxiety, depression, and restlessness. Although it induces sleep, night awakenings can still occur, so a restful night's sleep is not guaranteed. There is a long list of interacting drugs, and side effects include sedation, morning drowsiness, headache, cardiac problems, liver toxicity, and paradoxically, insomnia and excitability. Withdrawal symptoms may be seen with chronic use.

Kava (Piper mythysticum)

The extract of this plant has long been used by Pacific Islanders for reducing anxiety and enhancing relaxation. It is used today to treat benzodiazepene withdrawal, stress and anxiety, and short-term insomnia. Since its introduction to America in the 1980s, it has been used mostly as a drink additive, although the extract can be purchased as an herbal supplement. Studies show kava has a slight antianxiety effect. While it is generally safe, serious side effects have occasionally been reported. It was suspected of causing liver damage and was taken off the market in several countries but only carried a warning in America. After more study, this ceased to be a concern and the ban and warnings were lifted; however, several cases of liver damage could not be explained by any other mechanism, so caution is still recommended. Chronic use may depress the bone marrow. Minor side effects include headache, stomach complaints, fatigue, and restlessness. Kava interacts with a number of psychiatric medications, including the antipsychotics and anticonvulsants, so it should not be taken without your mental health professional's knowledge and consent.

Natural Endorphins Through Exercise

Regular exercise is important for overall good health, and exercising at the same time daily will help keep the body's internal clock synchronized. Aerobic exercise has a short-term antidepressant effect due to the natural endorphins that are released. Not only does exercise help lift mood, but it also helps counteract the weight gain bipolar meds often cause. There does not appear to be a long-term antidepressant effect from exercise, so it should not replace medication as treatment for depression. Patients on lithium should avoid excessive sweating, as lithium toxicity may result from the excessive sodium loss that sweating causes. While reports of lithium toxicity from heavy sweating are only anecdotal at this point and haven't been conclusively proven, it makes sense that a heavy sweater who doesn't replace electrolytes during exercise could potentially cause toxicity by upsetting the sodium level in the blood. It can't hurt to be careful and avoid exercising in very hot weather or in situations where heavy sweating might occur. Water aerobics in a pool with a temperature less than body temperature or exercising in a cool room or during the cool parts of the day may help avoid this potential complication.

Electroconvulsive Therapy (ECT)

This procedure evolved from seizure therapy to treat schizophrenia (psychosis) in the 1930s. The idea that eventually developed into ECT arose when a Hungarian psychiatrist, Ladislas von Meduna, observed that psychosis and epilepsy rarely occurred in the same patient, so he began to induce a grand mal seizure in patients suffering from psychosis. These patients usually felt better after one treatment, but it took multiple treatments to achieve remission in about half of the patients, with the remaining half showing improvement. The seizure "resets" the brain, much like rebooting a computer. Dr. Meduna's work caused a great deal of excitement in the field of psychiatry because schizophrenia was considered untreatable and incurable at that time (Shorter and Healy 34–43).

In 1938, two Italians, neurologist Cerletti and psychiatrist Bini, observed electrodes placed on the heads of pigs, causing seizure-like activity and unconsciousness before the pigs were butchered at a Rome slaughterhouse, and realized this technique might be a safer way to trigger therapeutic seizures in psychiatric patients. They began experimenting with dogs until electrode placement was perfected, but when they tried the technique on their first human patient, no seizure occurred. It took multiple attempts over two days before they were successful. This patient went on to have a series of electroshock treatments and recovered from his psychosis, although he relapsed some time later.

Today, ECT is used to treat prolonged and severe depression, including psychotic depression and catatonia or, less often, severe mania. It is used when medical treatment has failed or when a rapid mood switch is needed for the safety of the patient or others, as in extremely psychotic mania or deeply suicidal depression. It appears to be safer than increasing or adding medication in the elderly or in pregnant or nursing females. Treatments are given two to three times a week although twice weekly treatments appear to cause less memory loss than treatments three times a week, with the same clinical outcome. The number of treatments varies between 4 and 12 and depends on an individual's response. Once maximal improvement has been achieved, treatment is terminated. While the majority of patients respond to ECT, relapses are common and maintenance ECT is sometimes performed for those individuals who relapse quickly or who remain poorly responsive to medication.

A sedative and general anesthesia is given along with a paralyzing neuromuscular agent so muscular seizure activity is minimized, thus preventing muscle or bone damage. Ventilation is assisted, oxygen is given, and all vital signs are closely monitored. The major complications are heart arrhythmias or respiratory problems during anesthesia or the seizure itself, but the mortality rate is low and the same as for minor surgery (1 in 10,000 patients). ECT does not bring about a permanent cure, with a relapse rate the same it would normally be for the psychiatric illness. Nor does ECT replace bipolar medication, although anticonvulsants and benzodiazepenes are lowered or discontinued during treatment because of their antiseizure effect. All other bipolar medications can be safely continued, although those on lithium or high doses of the antidepressant buproprion (Wellbutrin) should be carefully monitored. The asthma drug theophylline, diuretics and oral hypoglycemic agents need to be withheld before ECT treatment but can be safely restarted afterward.

Like all treatments, there are side effects to contend with, such as headache and muscle pain immediately after the procedure. ECT causes memory loss, which is officially reported to be mild and transient, although patients insist this memory loss to be much worse than reported. Short-term memory loss stretches from the time before the procedure to after the procedure, but long-term memory loss can occur. While those memories may return in around 7 months, sometimes this loss is permanent. Cognitive problems are commonly seen soon after treatment and generally improve, but there is evidence that cognitive problems may persist and this appears to be related to treatment technique or scheduling. Newer machines, unilateral electrodes, and briefer electrical pulses have optimized results while minimizing memory loss and cognitive dysfunction. Individuals who need ECT are usually grateful for the option because they feel hopeless and completely at the mercy of their disease. They are willing to risk potential side effects, which they consider a reasonable trade-off when compared to their severe mania or unrelenting, suicidal depression.

Both Behrman and Fisher have benefited from electroshock therapy. Behrman decided to undergo this treatment when it appeared his bipolar was medication-resistant and he worsened to the point where he felt he would not survive his next severely psychotic episode. By the time he and his family chose ECT, they felt he had nothing left to lose. After his first treatment, Behrman commented: "Someone repaired my brain this morning.... I've never felt this way before. I've never felt this happy—or is it healthy? I feel incredibly different than I did pre–ECT, which was just an hour ago. Like the hard concrete that filled my brain has been liquefied and drained from my skull ... the manic depression that was cycloning in my head hours before is now sleeping like a baby" (226, 229). Fisher chose ECT therapy over suicide: "So, when weighing the choice between ECT and DOA, the decision is easy to make.... Electricity as opposed to game over. I decided to ride the lightning instead of extinguishing the light of life that had once shown out of my eyes. I kept my wick lit for my daughter, Billie, for my mother, my brother—for my entire family—and for each friend I've made with both hands, one heart, two moods" (14).

Repetitive Transcranial Magnetic Stimulation (rTMS)

This treatment method, which is FDA approved for medication-failed major depression, uses magnetic pulses to induce a weak electrical current in targeted areas of the brain in order to alter the polarization of the neuron membrane, affecting neuron excitability. Despite controversy in the past over the effectiveness of this treatment, a recent multicenter study showed improvement in 69 percent of individuals, with 45 percent achieving complete remission a year after treatment. Since half of ECT patients relapse within 6 months, it appears that rTMS may be almost as effective as ECT, at least for nonpsychotic depression, but the results might not be as impressive for psychotic bipolar depression. The procedure of rTMS is done in 5 half hour sessions every week for 6 weeks and may induce hypomania or mania, which can sometimes happen with ECT but is rare. There are no seizures, memory loss, or cognitive problems with this noninvasive method of treatment.

Deep Brain Stimulation (DBS)

This appears to be a safe and effective long-term treatment for depression that refuses to respond to medication. It is invasive, however, requiring the implantation of electrodes in the regions of the brain that control mood. Holes are drilled in the skull under local anesthesia and electrode placement is done with the patient awake in order to confirm proper placement. A battery powered generator (IPG, or brain pacemaker) is implanted under the skin of the upper chest or abdomen under general anesthesia and sends a small current that is delivered to the mood regions of the brain through the implanted brain electrodes. The IPG and electrodes are connected by an insulated wire that runs behind the ear under the skin of the neck.

Although this treatment is still considered experimental for bipolar disease and is waiting for FDA approval, it is already approved for use in movement disorders like Parkinson's disease, essential tremor, and dystonia. Complications include those of surgery and hardware failure. Common side effects include headache and worsening mood, including hypomania, depression and suicidal thoughts. Other psychiatric side effects, such as panic reaction, hallucinations, lack of inhibition and hypersexuality and cognitive and memory problems, may occur in a small number of cases. These may resolve once the electrical stimulation is adjusted or terminated.

Vagus Nerve Stimulation (VNS)

This therapy was originally designed to treat epilepsy and is now used to treat depression in those failing four medications and ECT treatment. It is FDA approved and endorsed by the American Psychiatric Association, although there is some controversy regarding whether this treatment is effective. An electronic pacer sends signals for a few seconds per minute to the brain via the left vagus nerve, which has less cardiac efferent fibers than the right vagus nerve, thus reducing cardiac arrhythmias. The mechanism of mood alteration isn't known but may involve altering levels of neurotransmitters, specifically norepinephrine and GABA. Since the vagus nerve (the 10th cranial nerve) contains both sensory and motor nerve fibers to and from the brain, side effects are from vagal nerve stimulation and include hoarseness, cough, sore throat, or swallowing difficulties, which appear to be related to laryngeal muscle spasm. Hoarseness is the most common side effect and, while it is usually mild, it is persistent. There may be snoring and mild to severe sleep apnea from episodic decreases in respiratory function. Hypomania and mania have been reported.

Light Therapy (Phototherapy, Heliotherapy)

This treatment is based on evidence in seasonal affective disorder that decreased light in the fall and winter can cause depression and increased light in the spring and summer can cause hypomania or mania. A phototherapy light box containing LED lights at 10,000 lux or lower intensity of blue or green light at 350 lux is used within 1 hour of arising in the morning, for 30–90 minutes a day. Most of the eye and skin damaging UV rays have been filtered out. The lights need only reach the retina of the eyes, so the light box can be in front of the individual or slightly off to one side, and preferably the lights should be slightly above the eyes to prevent glare. Since the individual need only face the light box and not look directly at the lights, she can read, do computer work, or perform any other sedentary activity that allows her to stay in front of the light box for the prescribed time. It is important for the doctor to prescribe the amount of phototherapy each individual needs and to monitor each person for potential hypomania. Light therapy works for depression even in the absence of seasonal affective disorder, and can be used with or without antidepressants. Hypomania may be triggered and reproductive hormones may be stimulated. Individuals on drugs or herbs, such as St. John's wort, that cause photosensitivity or those that have porphyria or are on medications that may elicit porphyria, should not use light therapy.

Hospitalization

A mental hospitalization may be necessary on occasion when bipolar disease becomes unmanageable and requires intensive treatment. There are several scenarios where this might be necessary. The classic reason for committing someone involuntarily to a mental hospital is when they are a danger to themselves or others. While this usually implies suicidal thoughts or actions, the danger of self harm or harm to others is often higher during severe mania than during severe depression. The severely manic person doesn't usually intend to harm themselves or anyone else, but a marked lack of inhibition and impulse control along with severely impaired judgment or psychotic delusions of grandeur may lead to dangerous behavior that can kill or maim. Extreme paranoia may bring about violent and aggressive behavior that may harm others as well as the bipolar. Certainly those who have had previous suicide attempts or who have access to the means to kill themselves, those who live alone, those who have a history of violence or impulsive behaviors, those who are so depressed they feel hopeless, or those who suffer substance abuse are at high risk for suicide and would be more likely to be hospitalized during an acute mood attack. Severe depression that leaves an individual unable to care for himself requires hospitalization as well.

Hospitalization allows for rapid calming of an agitated manic patient and intensive adjustment of medications that would have to occur more gradually on an outpatient basis. Side effects and medication response can be monitored under the watchful eyes of the hospital professionals. Doses can be rapidly increased (or decreased) and drugs changed without the responsibilities and stresses of regular life to consider. Without worrying about driving or the responsibilities of work, school, or caring for children, sedation or other side effects that would interfere in the functioning of normal life can be tolerated in the hospital setting.

It may take 4 weeks or longer to stabilize an acute attack and a switch to the opposite mood state may occur once the acute mood state resolves. Partial hospitalization, when an individual spends days in the hospital setting but goes home at night, may bridge the gap between hospitalization and discharge, but there must be a stable home environment and a supportive family at home every night for this option to succeed. Outpatient treatment can also serve as a bridge from hospital care to normal life. Education about bipolar disease, medication monitoring, and psychotherapy are some of the services that are available on an outpatient basis and will help ease the transition back to normal life.

Summary

1. Individuals on lithium must keep their salt intake stable to avoid altering their lithium blood levels.
2. The atypical antipsychotics can cause metabolic syndrome, so a diet low in simple sugars and starches with healthy fats is recommended.
3. A standard daily dose of fish oil (omega–3 fatty acids) may help psychotic patients.

4. A deficiency of any of the B complex vitamins, other than B12, is rare in this country, so standard daily doses probably aren't needed but won't do any harm.

5. There are a number of herbal preparations, many of which interfere with bipolar or other medications and should be taken only under the supervision of a mental health professional.

6. Exercise has a mild antidepressant effect and will help counteract the weight gain that accompanies many of the bipolar medications.

7. Electroconvulsive therapy is effective and often lifesaving but is reserved for cases of severe depression or mania that are unresponsive to medical treatment.

8. There are several brain stimulation techniques (rTMS, DBS, VNS) but none work as well as ECT, although rTMS appears promising.

9. Light therapy is useful in the treatment of depression but can trigger hypomania or mania.

10. Hospitalization is necessary when intensive treatment or protection is needed.

Chapter 12

The Dark Side of Bipolar Disease

Bipolar is a serious disease, and while it can be treated successfully in most cases, it should never be forgotten that the disease can be fatal, especially early in its course before effective treatment has been worked out and before the bipolar is ready to do the hard work of recovery. While creativity and genius enhance the lives of some bipolars, psychosis afflicts others, and nearly all bipolars have some degree of delusional thinking during certain mood states. Hypomania is pleasurable in the beginning when the bipolar is full of confidence and energy, driving the urge to engage in goal-oriented activities. A continued rise in mood slowly begins to unravel organization, continuity, and thought processes so that function begins to decline. As hypomania approaches mania, delusions become more extreme and the bipolar's beliefs may become outrageous. If psychosis occurs, the bipolar cannot distinguish between reality and non-reality and the delusions will reflect this shift in perception. While nearly all bipolars suffer some degree of delusional thinking, not every bipolar will have psychotic thinking, frank psychosis, or hallucinations.

Suicide is strikingly common in bipolar disease and most suicides occur in the mixed or depressed mood states. This is the elephant in the room, the dreaded topic that no one wants to talk about but has to be acknowledged and accepted and not swept under the rug. Suicidal thinking is so common in depression that it is one of the criteria for diagnosis. To pretend it doesn't occur is simply denial, with the potential for life-threatening consequences. Bipolar disease can be fatal, from accidental death during mania to suicide during depression or mixed attacks; those are the facts. If you ever begin to have suicidal thoughts, you must be honest with your mental health professional or doctor in order to get appropriate treatment. Sadly, you can't always depend on the medical profession to detect your depression or suicidal thinking without your help.

Delusions, Psychoses, and Hallucinations

When a person can't distinguish what's real from what's not real, they are said to be delusional or psychotic, depending on the severity of their break from reality. The difference between delusional thinking and frank psychosis is simply a matter of degree. A delusion is a false belief representing only a break from reality, but this belief is very real to the delusional person and may or may not impair functioning. Psychosis, on the other hand, represents a more complete break from reality and functioning is usually impaired. This can be very alarming to others who aren't aware of the delusional thinking that lies behind strikingly odd or strange behavior. Behrman describes psychosis like this: "In my most psychotic stages, I imagine myself chewing on sidewalks and buildings, swallowing sunlight and clouds" (xix). Even the most supportive family and friends sometimes cannot deal with an acutely psychotic loved one for any extended period of time due to the constant stress and fear that the psychotic bipolar will hurt herself or others. Vonnegut agrees: "The psychotic state is a destructive process. A fire can't burn that brightly without melting circuits.... Fixed delusions, fears, loss of flexibility, loss of concrete thinking, and low stress tolerance make relationships, jobs, and family next to impossible and then impossible" (7).

In the not too distant past, it was believed that delusions and psychosis were seen only in schizophrenia and many bipolars were misdiagnosed. I have a family member who carried the schizophrenia diagnosis for years until the correct diagnosis of bipolar disease was made. Since then, it has been discovered that delusional and psychotic manias appear to run in families and are most often seen in bipolar-I. The earlier the age of onset of bipolar, the more likely a person will have psychosis. After many studies it was determined that thought processes were disrupted in both schizophrenics and manic bipolars but that the type of thought disruption differs in each. Manics tend to have more complex speech with disorderly thought *structure*, while schizophrenics tend to have less complex speech and disorderly thought *content*. Disordered thinking tends to be reversible in bipolar disease, while it remains more chronic in schizophrenics. It appears that there may be a common genetic susceptibility linking delusional thinking, psychosis, and bipolar disease and that bipolar disease and schizophrenia may share these particular susceptibility genes.

Delusions

Delusions usually match the mood state a person is in. During mania, delusions are frequently grandiose and wish-fulfilling or mystical and religious, but they can sometimes be paranoid and violent. For example, the bipolar may entertain delusions about having special powers or may believe they have been chosen for an important mission or that a special secret of the universe will be revealed to them. They may feel as if they can walk through traffic without harm or fly off tall buildings. The people on the TV may be talking just to them, money found on the street has been left just for them, parking spaces open up magically as soon as they arrive, and everything in the world is centered on them and them alone. As Mark Vonnegut describes it, "Thoughts come into the mind as firmly established truth.... The fantastic presents itself as fact" (105).

If the manic mood state becomes mixed or agitated, paranoia may set in and the delusions that follow will usually reflect that mindset. Danger lurks around every corner, strangers making eye contact signal a conspiracy, and food or air is harmful or poisoned. Delusions during depression may take the form of somatic complaints (hypochondria) in which a hidden illness is suspected or minor physical symptoms are blown out of proportion or thought to represent a disastrous disease. A person may go from doctor to doctor, chasing vague complaints, convinced that something is terribly wrong and while it may be recognized the person is a hypochondriac, the delusional nature of their somatic complaints may go unrecognized.

Melissa McCarter was hospitalized during a psychotic manic episode and she describes her delusions as differing only in degree: "My delusions, perhaps, are more elaborate than the day to day delusions that anybody has to function sanely" (492–96). McCarter believed fried chicken served for lunch at the hospital one day was actually fried human heart and she was unable to eat. When asked by a still-hungry fellow patient if he could have her chicken, McCarter's delusion vanished and she was able to eat her food without difficulty. Delusions during mania can wax and wane along with fluctuations of the mood state. McCarter eventually learned to live with her delusions, which never completely disappeared: "This, I am coming to believe, is the dividing line between sanity and insanity—only keeping the delusions that serve life, and letting go of the ones that create a certain stuckness and immobility" (504–8).

Psychosis

A psychotic brain is a confused brain that can no longer distinguish information that it has manufactured from within itself from sensory information coming from outside itself. It is overwhelmed with stimuli, both internal and external, as it becomes flooded with both false and true information. All filtering mechanisms disappear as senses and emotions become intense and powerful. Dr. Sis describes one of her psychotic states like this:

I believe that all the bright lights and singing birds I saw and heard were absolutely real. These things are really there and other people can't see or hear them, until their "defenses" are down. I saw auras around every star and every streetlight. Lights shimmered and became intensely brighter as I watched them. I wandered all over one night, from one bright light to another.

Hornbacher describes the shift from mania to madness to psychosis like this:

Madness will push you anywhere it wants. It never tells you where you're going, or why. It dangles something sparkly before you, shimmering like that water patch on the road up ahead. You will drive around until you find it, the treasure, the thing you most desire. You will never find it. Madness may mock you so long you will die of the search. Or it will tire of you, turn its back, oblivious as you go flying ... But at first, as always, it fools me. At first it is lovely, showy, hallucinatory, neon bright. I am viscerally, violently alive. I don't know when I turn the corner from merely crazy to completely psychotic.... [W]e draw into ourselves, our eyes rolling back in our heads so that soon we can see nothing but the chaos and terror of our own minds" (114).

As you can tell from these descriptions of psychotic states, most bipolars, even when psychotic, remain at least partly aware of where they are and who they are unless they are extremely psychotic. Their memories generally remain intact and in hypomania and mania may even be enhanced. In the extremes of depression or mania, however, severe distractibility and difficulty concentrating adversely affect memory. We have been led to believe that being "crazy" means becoming someone completely different from the person we were before. Even the term "break" as used in "psychotic break" or "break from reality" seems to imply a break so complete it changes who the person normally is. A psychotic or extremely delusional person can certainly seem that way to friends and family. While that may be true in extreme cases, a bipolar person can lose his grip on reality without completely letting go of sanity. He may still be capable of functioning on some level while hearing voices or entertaining delusions. While many lack full insight into what is happening, they may still be aware that they need help and a few may even be able to get help for themselves.

When Mark Vonnegut was hospitalized after trying to throw himself out the third-story window of his home, he was taken to the hospital where he was on faculty. He was partially dressed, acutely psychotic, and restrained on a gurney in a hallway as he waited to be admitted. As people passed by, he told them not to worry as he explained that the police had overreacted and as soon as his doctor arrived everything would be straightened out. He wondered why he had been taken to a hospital where he was so well known and why he hadn't been allowed to dress completely and why they couldn't have respected his privacy enough to place him in a room rather than in a public hallway. As psychotic as he was, he was still thinking clearly enough to be aware of these very normal, humiliating things. Eventually he saw a nurse he knew and naturally she was shocked to see this prominent doctor restrained and in a state of undress. As she tried to hold back her tears, Vonnegut reassured her that everything was going to be okay. Even in the vast ocean of psychosis, there are, thankfully, welcome islands of sanity.

Vonnegut was so delusional and psychotic that, while hospitalized, he thought he was in a battle to avoid nuclear war and to bring down the Berlin wall and that he had been chosen, over everyone else in America, because of his faith and problem-solving abilities. He believed he was being smuggled to various countries concealed in layers of cotton and foam, where he would battle their craziest person and be judged on the basis of depth of feeling. Mark won every battle. When he got to China, they conceded, saying they didn't have anyone as crazy as he was. The final showdown was the Russian Bear. By the time he was ready for this battle, his psychosis lifted and he saw that his battles were actually against a group of teenage girl bullies on the psych ward who threw things at him and taunted him. The leader of the pack was an overweight, curly-haired girl—his Russian Bear. Vonnegut, a middle-aged pediatrician, stood up to her. She dissolved in tears, and that was the end of his elaborate psychotic delusion. Perhaps his sensation of being wrapped in cotton and foam had been at times when he was restrained, either medically or physically, on the ward. Even when he was extremely psychotic, he was still reacting to what was going on around him, although his interpretation of what was happening outside his brain was altered by his psychotic delusions.

Eventually, the ability to maintain coherent thought, to form concepts or abstract ideas, or to express thought decreases as brain function deteriorates. In severe manic psychosis, speech may deteriorate into disjointed, detached words or phrases that make no sense to the listener as thoughts become increasingly disordered. At this point, the severely psychotic person is unable to communicate through language and "speaking in tongues" may occur. Virginia Woolf's husband described manic periods when Woolf's thinking and speech would deteriorate so that she would talk nonstop for days (pressure of speech), paying no attention to anything going on around her. At first Virginia's husband could understand what she was saying; but after a day or so, she lapsed into nothing more than a string of disconnected words. Eventually she would collapse in exhaustion, silent at last.

Hallucinations

Hallucinations occur in three-fourths of manic episodes and are more common in the psychotic state than they are in delusional thinking. They can be categorized according to the five senses—auditory (hearing), visual (sight), taste, olfactory (smell), and tactile (touch)—and represent the brain's inability to distinguish sensory stimulation coming from outside the body from information originating in the brain itself. Women seem to have more hallucinations, particularly visual and auditory hallucinations, than men, but that might be because women tend to report their hallucinations more often than men. Reclusive women seem to experience both types of hallucinations more frequently than more sociable, less reclusive women.

Auditory hallucinations are the most common type of hallucination reported and occur when voices are heard but no one is around. They usually occur at night and when the bipolar is alone. Sometimes these voices may come from a visual hallucination (Mrs. Mamone's dead mother, for example), animals speaking to people, inanimate objects (Mrs. Mamone's sculpture) or inside a person's head (God talking to the bipolar). Depending on the mood state, these voices may be comforting or neutral, although they can sometimes be accusatory. They may tell the bipolar to do something or they may be cautionary or critical of the person to the point of torture. The voice may come from someone the person recognizes, like a dead family member, or a religious figure such as God, Jesus, or Satan.

Mark Vonnegut, after years of steady but not excessive use, stopped his moderate drinking and Xanax at bedtime and suffered his first psychotic break in nearly 15 years. As he was praying to God to help him get through either alcohol or, more likely, benzodiazepene withdrawal, he suddenly began to hear God talking to him, assuring him that he would be okay. As Vonnegut became more psychotic, the voices that had come to him in previous psychotic attacks told him the world was ending and its fate was in his hands. The voices told him exactly what he needed to do in order to save the world, but first he had to prove himself faithful and unselfish enough to be the savior of the world. He was instructed to jump out of a closed third-story window in his home. God assured him he would be unharmed and if he did this one thing the agitation and the voices telling him to do even worse things would stop. He missed the window, although he hit close enough to send the frame and glass flying to the ground below. Vonnegut's auditory hallucinations drove him not to kill himself, as it might seem to others, but to prove his faith; God's voice was comforting and Mark felt very special to have been chosen for God's mission.

Visual hallucinations are the second most common hallucination to occur and a person sees things that aren't there, usually as a brief illusion rather than a fully formed image. They are frequently religious in nature, as Dr. Sis describes: "I remember a vision of a bright white angel—for years I have called him Mr. Clean. He looked just like that. He was very real." William

Blake, the English Romantic poet who suffered the great highs and deep depressions that are typical of bipolar disorder, experienced hallucinations and delusions, believing that he spoke to spirits that surrounded him. His psychotic visions clearly inspired his art. Percy Bysshe Shelley, yet another British Romantic poet who appears to have suffered from bipolar disorder with psychotic hallucinations, once claimed that he saw a baby clapping its hands while rising out of the ocean. Those with visual hallucinations may feel special and chosen and may not wish to share their vision with anyone. Dr. Sis relates a visual and auditory hallucination during a psychotic attack:

> That Christmas I sat on the couch for either 1 day or 2 days. No food, no water, no urination. I got really dehydrated and my meds were either too low (I couldn't tell if I had taken them or not) or so concentrated from my dehydration that I was delirious. I subsequently had severe chest pain and I think I had a heart attack. But the whole time I was watching TV and every damn thing was funny. Even the commercials were hilarious. Then the Christian programs came on. Here's where it got strange. The one they call the 500 Club had Pat Robertson's son on there. I usually turn that stuff off immediately. This time they were all holding hands and praying for somebody. This time it was me. You know how everybody has always stumbled over my name.... Well, this guy started praying for someone who was "in great pain on this Christmas Eve." He said her name was [Dr. Sis wrote the mispronunciation of her name], then no, it's [she wrote her correct name]. I jumped up off the couch. He then went forth to name everything that was wrong with me on that night. Severe chest pains, a lump in my cervical spine and even a damn rash on my face. The list went on. He talked about my abnormal separation from my family.... [I]t was spooky. He called me by name and my name is totally unique. So this is another "psychotic" experience where the TV people are talking about me.

Hallucinations involving taste are usually unpleasant, as are olfactory hallucinations. Food may smell and taste "off" or tainted, and if paranoia exists poisoning may be suspected. Tactile hallucinations may involve the sensation of crawling bugs or other unpleasant experiences. These hallucinations may not be very obvious to others. A young girl who picks at her plate of food may seem to be watching her figure or perhaps be a picky eater when she actually believes her food smells or tastes spoiled, even if others around her are eating the same food without any problem. Others with auditory hallucinations, particularly if they are the religious type, may go unnoticed for a time, as phrases like "talking to God" are commonly used and are not meant as literally as those with auditory hallucinations mean them. Like Mrs. Mamone from chapter 1, bipolars with hallucinations (and delusions) may not choose to share them with everyone, or they may assume that everyone sees, hears, tastes or feels what they do.

Suicide

I once did a survey of all the primary medical practices in the community where I live, which has one of highest suicide rates in our state, to see how many of them screened for depression, because so many patient physical complaints stem from depression rather than from real physical problems. Only one practice did depression screening. I also found that almost no practice, even the one that screened for depression, asked about suicidal thoughts if depression was diagnosed, and there was little to no follow-up if a person was placed on an antidepressant. This means no one was specifically looking for and asking about suicide risk factors, such as previous suicide attempts, anxiety, agitation, or substance abuse.

Unfortunately, this is more common that you would suspect. Studies have shown that, while almost half of suicidal patients see their doctors within a month of their suicide and 20 percent see a mental health professional (Luoma, Martin, and Pearson), very few directly communicate their suicidal feelings to their doctors. To get treatment for depression in my community and many others, an individual needs to be proactive and talk openly about feeling depressed or suicidal. While some individuals are able to do this, many can't bring themselves to admit they need help and others aren't aware their physical complaints stem from depression. The very nature of depression prevents most people from seeing a doctor in the first place; and if they get the energy to actually show up, it's not surprising they have no further motivation to ask for the help they need. Therefore, it is the responsibility of the doctor or mental health professional to make the next move.

The majority of individuals who commit suicide (90–95 percent) suffer from some form of psychiatric illness, most commonly bipolar disease or severe depression. Bipolars commit suicide at an alarmingly high rate and are fifteen times more likely to kill themselves than the general population (Jamison, *Night Falls Fast* 101–2). Untreated, partially treated, treatment-resistant, and newly diagnosed bipolars or those with substance abuse are more likely to self harm. The risk of suicide is highest during a mixed mood state, where depression and mania are combined and agitation is present, with a severely depressed mood state running a close second. While statistics appear to show that suicide is more common in severe non-bipolar depression rather than bipolar disease, a significant number of those depressions are now thought to be bipolar depressions, specifically bipolar-II. If we expand the definition of bipolar disease to include highly recurrent depressions, the statistics for suicide under the bipolar heading increase over that of non-bipolar depression. While one in five individuals with severe non-bipolar depression may attempt suicide, studies have shown that up to half of severely depressed bipolars will attempt suicide (Jamison, *Night Falls Fast* 110). These bipolars often have more severe depression with a mixed, agitated component as compared to those who suffer from non-bipolar depression. This results in a greater intent to die, which leads to a more detailed suicide plan, a more serious suicide attempt and a higher incidence of completed suicide. Overall, more women than men attempt suicide and survive, and more men succeed at their suicide attempts (they choose more lethal means of self harm). The suicide rate for men and women is about equal in bipolar disease or even slightly less for men. Bipolar is potentially a lethal disease.

Just as there is often a seasonal component to bipolar mood swings, there can be a seasonal component to bipolar suicide. The highest peak appears to be in late spring and early summer, with another, smaller peak in October. This appears to correlate with hours of bright sunshine during the day and not with the length of day. Aggressive behavior, which translates into putting a suicidal plan into action, peaks in late spring and early summer in both men and women, when winter depression transitions to a mixed state as mood begins to rise again. The October peak can be explained by a post-manic drop in mood or a mixed state after a summer manic or hypomanic state.

Suicides often cluster in families, and if an individual has other family members who have committed suicide, her risk of also committing suicide is five-fold greater than if the family didn't have this history (Baldessarini and Hennen). This implies a genetic component to suicide that has been confirmed by twin studies. Identical twins have an increased risk of suicide over fraternal twins, and fraternal twins also carry an increased risk for suicide because of their family history but not as much as identical twins. Children adopted into bipolar families do not show an increased risk of suicide. Ernest Hemingway's family was full of suicides over multiple generations. I know a family with 4 bipolar suicides (that I'm aware of) over 3 generations. Another family had multiple suicides over several past generations with only a bipolar spectrum presentation (stable hypomania with aggressive outbursts from time to time) in the current generation and no suicides (yet) in the past two generations. At this time it is not known what trait is inherited that makes an individual more likely than another to commit suicide. This "suicide gene" may code for impulsivity, aggression, violence, or some other trait that makes it more likely to self-harm.

"I had been in a desperate depression, so bleak, so utterly hopeless that killing myself seemed the only solution that made any sense. Night after night I dreamed about suicide" (Cheney 178). This is how Cheney describes her suicidal depression, a mental state that seems so hopeless that dying appeared the only way out. Suicide is not really about killing oneself but about ending the pain and suffering, which seems endless to the sufferer. If a severely depressed bipolar doesn't see any way out of what appears to be an endless depression, dying becomes the only solution to the never-ending suffering. Anxiety and agitation simply add to the misery, and substance abuse piles on yet another layer of suffering, creating a crater that appears too deep to escape from. Fisher explains severe bipolar depression this way: "That's what can take simple sadness and turn it into sadness squared. It's what revs up the motor of misery, guns the engine of an unpleasant experience, filling it with rocket fuel and blasting into a place in the stratosphere that is oh-so-near to something like a suicidal tendency—a place where the wish to continue living in this painful place is all but completely absent" (13–14).

I learned a wonderful representational model of suicide at a suicide conference I once attended. Suicidal thoughts are depicted as a fast-moving river that pours over a precipice as a waterfall, which represents the final act of suicide. An individual standing on the bank of this river, dipping a toe into the water, may be having a passing thought about suicide but isn't going to do anything active to bring it about. Once an individual steps into the water, suicidal thinking is more serious, but as long as this person stays near the bank, the current is weak and suicide isn't likely. The closer a person moves toward the middle of the river where the current is strong, the more likely suicide becomes. Once an individual gets to the middle of the river, the current is so strong that being swept over the edge is inevitable. Intervention to prevent suicide is possible at all stages except for this last stage, when the current is too strong for rescue to occur. The closer to the riverbank, where the current is weaker, the more likely we are to save a person from self-harm. The point of this model is to teach us the importance of identifying suicidal individuals before they have waded to the center of the river where they will be swept away, regardless of our attempts to save them.

It's extremely common in severe bipolar depression or mixed states to wade into suicidal waters, so what keeps bipolars close to the bank rather than going to the center of the river where they will be swept over the edge? Connections with family and friends who love and depend on the bipolar and a good support system—professional and otherwise—go a long way toward keeping these suffering individuals around. The courage to ask for help, coping strategies, religious beliefs, and the knowledge that no matter how endless the current mood state seems to be, it, too, shall pass, also help make survival more likely. As Cheney says, "The cruelest curse of the disease is also its most sacred promise: You will not feel this way forever" (76).

Your mental health professional is trained to assess suicidal risk and act to protect you if she feels you are at risk for self-harm. You need to be honest about your feelings and tell the truth about the suicidal thoughts or feelings you are having. Some bipolars are honest with their family members yet deny their feelings or intentions when their mental health professional inquires about them. Perhaps they think nothing can be done to help or they are embarrassed to admit how desperate they feel. Even if you think nothing can be done to alter your mood state, there are therapeutic options available to help alleviate your suffering, sometimes in a hospital setting and sometimes in an outpatient setting, depending on your risk level. Even if you think being hospitalized represents a failure in your control over your disease, it's an important and sometimes necessary way to keep you safe and help you recover.

If you believe the world might be better off without you, I assure you that your friends and family will strongly disagree with you. I've never seen a suicide where the family was relieved or happy their loved one was gone, no matter how much trouble they caused their family. Suicide leaves behind a legacy of incredible pain, suffering, and guilt. Your loved ones will be left devastated, forever wondering why you didn't come to them for help, no matter how complicated your history with them may have been. The grieving after the suicide of a loved one is complicated and prolonged. Even if you feel you have no self worth when you are in the throes of severe depression, your friends and family do not feel this way about you. No one will ever take your place in their lives.

Summary

1. Bipolar is a serious yet treatable disease, but it is sometimes fatal before treatment is optimized.
2. A delusion is a false belief representing only a mild break from reality; functioning may or may not be impaired.
3. Delusions match the mood state in which they occur; in hypomania or mania they may be grandiose, religious, or wish-fulfilling, but when mania becomes mixed, they may become paranoid or hypochondriacal.
4. Psychosis represents a more marked departure from reality, and functioning is nearly always impaired.
5. The psychotic brain cannot distinguish between sensory input from outside the brain and input coming from inside the brain.
6. Hallucinations are very common in manic episodes and in advanced psychosis.
7. Most hallucinations are auditory and are usually comforting or neutral in tone, although some can be accusatory; visual hallucinations are usually a brief illusion rather than a fully formed image.
8. Suicide is most common in the depressed or mixed mood states.
9. Some bipolar families show multiple suicides over generations, suggesting a genetic component.
10. No matter how hopeless or endless a suicidal depression seems, it will always switch to another mood state eventually.

Chapter 13

The Bipolar Edge

Genius and "madness" have been linked since ancient times, and for good reason, but is there really a bipolar "edge" when it comes to creativity and genius? In my own family, two bipolar members are extremely creative, one demonstrating incredible intellectual, artistic, and musical abilities from a very early age. The third member never finished high school, had severe social anxiety, worked in a factory until psychosis and substance abuse took their toll, and is now chronically and profoundly mentally ill. Not all exceptional people are bipolar and not all bipolar people are exceptional. How is it possible for one bipolar to be full of prodigious ability while another barely scrapes by?

Bipolar disease afflicts all sorts of people, some of whom are born with their own unique set of talents and abilities based on their specific family genetics. The increased energy and enhanced functioning that accompany hypomania and early mania magnify whatever personal traits and abilities an individual possesses from birth. If a person is genetically blessed with high intelligence or artistic or musical talent, those inherent abilities will be magnified during hypomania, when ideas flow and when motivation to work and create is high. A person less endowed with special abilities may spend hypomanic times energetically cleaning house, cutting the grass, or building a shed in the backyard. These people may or may not be creative—there are creative ways to clean house, cut grass, or build a shed—but they will actively pursue their nonartistic or nonintellectual interests in an enhanced manner when hypomanic.

Bipolar individuals blessed with a rich, creative inheritance or intellectual ability are frequently raised in a stimulating (and possibly bipolar spectrum) home environment where such creative or intellectual pursuits are encouraged and praised. It has been argued, then, that because these children are brought up in a creative environment, they choose creative careers due to the creative pursuits they were exposed to by their parents. But creative families produce a wide range of creative offspring with many creative professions represented.

182

A child raised in a literary home, for example, may grow up to be an artist or a musician but may have never been exposed to those particular creative fields while growing up. Does this creativity come from a stimulating and creative home environment or does it come from the bipolar disease itself?

Not all bipolars are creative, although many are. And there are certainly plenty of creative non-bipolar individuals who may also be eccentric, energetic, or even a bit moody. Many, if not most, creative types will not manifest any significant mood disorder during their lifetimes. Creativity does not always equal bipolarity, and bipolarity does not always equal creativity.

Genius

Originally, the word "genius" was used to describe a brilliantly creative individual with "God-given" or "divine" artistic talent and ability. Eventually the word generalized to include those with special intellectual as well as artistic abilities, whether musical, literary, or visual arts, and only later did the term "creativity" come to describe mostly artistic individuals, leaving the "genius" label more firmly attached to highly functioning intellectual types. That being said, there remains some crossover in usage, with the term "genius" used for particularly brilliant artistic creators and the term "creative" used for particularly novel and fresh intellectual insights.

Lewis Terman began a study in 1921 (Andreasen, *Creating Brain* 12–13) to determine if creativity and high intelligence were equal. He followed a group of schoolchildren with high IQ scores throughout their lifetimes and did not find a high level of creativity in that group, although most grew up to be successful adults with careers that ranged from the professional vocations to semiskilled labor. A few of the individuals were indeed creative (Robert Oppenheimer was a notable example, but he was also bipolar), and a few more had creative interests outside their professions. The majority of these high-IQ individuals were not creative. While some level of intelligence is most likely required for an individual to make full use of their creativity, creativity appears to be a separate and distinct mental ability that is not bound to high IQ.

Creativity

How do we differentiate an extraordinarily creative person from someone with ordinary creativity? Some of the most important characteristics are curiosity and the ability to respond to the world in an open and inquisitive manner and to make new connections and have new ideas based on observations not bound by convention or habit. The world is never black or white for the creative individual but is instead experienced in shades of gray. Ideas come from such flexibility and the ability to observe the world in an open-ended manner, leading to originality of thought. A creative person doesn't just notice the bird looking for scraps of food on the pavement and think "there's a bird looking for scraps of food on the ground." If they are the scientific type, they notice the behavior of the bird as it struts around or cocks its head. They will evaluate the shape of the body or beak or wing and notice what type of food the bird prefers and how it goes about looking for it. The artistic type might notice the shifting colors as sunlight reflects off the feathers or appreciate the shape-shifting of the bird's shadow as it moves about, while the musical type may delight in the cadences of its birdsong. The poetic type may notice the beauty of the bird's movement or appearance and respond emotionally to what the bird appears to represent at that moment in time.

Ideas flow, connections are made, thoughts expand, and a simple bird on the ground searching for food may serve as the inspiration for a scientific principle, artwork, a poem, or a work of music. Associations are made that may have had little to do, in the end, with the actual bird, as these free-form associations are linked with other ideas, feelings, emotions, and concepts in the extraordinarily creative person's brain. Call these associative links insights or inspirations, if you will, but they are simply by-products of the creative person's ability to free-associate facts, experiences, or ideas in such a manner that they become connected in novel and original ways. The creative person is rarely bored; inspiration is everywhere.

Genius, Creativity, and Bipolarity

The connection between genius, creativity and "madness" has been noted for thousands of years and many studies have been done in the past century to determine whether nature versus nurture is responsible. Creativity was first linked to psychosis and that link has held up over time. Although this was originally attributed to schizophrenia, now that we can differentiate between the two mental illnesses associated with psychosis (schizophrenia and bipolar), it has become clear that creativity is most strongly linked to mood disorders, mainly bipolar disease. And while studies support a link between creativity and bipolar, in both patients and their non-bipolar family members, that exact link remains unknown, although researchers are getting closer to pinning down the genetics of bipolar, schizophrenia, and creativity itself.

Some non-bipolar family members in a bipolar family also exhibit creativity. Perhaps they inherited this trait separately from the bipolar or they may have a subthreshold or nonclinical bipolar spectrum manifestation of the disease, where the creativity is expressed but not the bipolarity. The more we learn about the bipolar spectrum, the more we suspect that creativity in the absence of bipolarity, in a bipolar family, most likely represents subthreshold or nonclinical "disease." Conversely, creative folk have a higher than average rate of mood disorders when compared to the general population. Case history studies of geniuses conducted in the late 1800s and early 1900s revealed a higher rate of mental illness—particularly manic-depression and "insanity"— in artistic geniuses as compared to nonartistic geniuses, such as those in scientific fields. Of even more interest was the discovery that first degree relatives of these artistic geniuses had higher than average rates of mental illness, ranging from mild mood disorders to full-blown manic-depression to suicide, suggesting the concept of a spectrum of presentations of bipolar disease.

The often quoted Iowa Writer's Workshop study (Andreasen, "Creativity and Mental Illness") revealed an 80 percent lifetime incidence of a mood disorder episode in the 30 writers studied compared to a 30 percent incidence in the 30 nonwriters of the control group. While only 10 percent of the nonwriters had a diagnosis of manic-depression, 43 percent of the writers carried that diagnosis. There was a 37 percent incidence of severe depression in the writer's group compared to 17 percent in the control group and 30 percent in the writer's group suffered from alcoholism compared to 7 percent in the control group. A 7 percent suicide rate was seen in the writer's group with no suicides in the control group, although this finding was not considered to be statistically significant.

A study of prominent current British writers and artists (Jamison, "Mood Disorders") showed that around a third of the group, mostly the artists and playwrights, reported severe mood swings, while a fourth, mostly the poets and novelists, had experienced periods of hypomania or mania. Only biographers reported no mood swings or heightened mood states. All (100 percent) of the poets, novelists, and artists described extremely creative periods symptomatic of hypomania, while 88 percent of the playwrights and only 20 percent of the biographers did so. These creative periods lasted on average 1 to 4 weeks but ranged from a day to a month in length and were preceded in 55 percent of the subjects by a sudden uplifting of mood. Over a quarter of the subjects reported irritability, restlessness, and anxiety as well as distress, paranoia, and suicidal feelings prior to the onset of their creative period. Slightly less than a third experienced a mixed mood state of both increased and decreased mood. Nearly all the subjects, particularly the poets, felt their intense moods were vital both to their art and creative process.

An Icelandic study (Karlsson) revealed that both psychotic patients and their first degree relatives were more likely to be accomplished in either the artistic or academic fields and, surprisingly, it showed an increased risk of mental illness in accomplished scholars and their families. Later review of study data showed a strong correlation between mood disorders (especially bipolar) and creativity. The McNeil twin study (McNeil) was designed to clarify the question of whether a genetic or environmental influence was responsible for the clustering of creativity and bipolar disease in some families. The result clearly demonstrated what McNeil called a "prebirth factor," in that rate and type of mental illness in adults who were adopted soon after birth were more likely to correlate with the biological parents than with the adoptive parents. This correlation was strongest in highly creative adults and their biological parents. There was no correlation between mental illness in the adoptive parents and the creativity of the adopted adults. For example, 30 percent of the highly creative adopted adults suffered from mental illness, along with 27.7 percent of their biological parents, while only 5.3 percent of their adoptive parents suffered from a mental illness. This implies a genetic inheritance for both creativity and mental illness.

A Harvard study (Richards, Kinney, and Lunde) hypothesized that genetic vulnerability to manic-depression might be accompanied by a predisposition to creativity. Bipolar and cyclothymic patients and their first degree relatives were compared to a control group. Results showed that creativity was increased in the bipolars, cyclothymes and their relatives. Among the bipolar group, however, the normal relatives and cyclothymes scored higher in creativity than the bipolars. The cyclothymes and normal relatives were close, though, with the normal relatives scoring only slightly higher. Whether the normal relatives are truly normal or have a subclinical expression of bipolar vulnerability was not known at the time.

A recent study (MacCabe) shows a strong correlation between bipolar disease and high academic performance, particularly in creative subjects such as the humanities as opposed to the sciences. This correlation showed that academically talented teens, particularly boys, were nearly four times as likely to develop bipolar disease by the time they were 26 as compared to their more academically normal peers. Interestingly, low academic performance was associated with a moderately increased risk of bipolar disease. This study supports the widely held belief that exceptional intellectual ability, particularly in the more creative academic subjects, is linked to bipolar disease.

A recent Swedish study (Kyaga, Liechtenstein, and Boman) of 300,000 schizophrenics, bipolars, and unipolar depressives and their first degree relatives explored whether creativity was linked to mental illness. The researchers looked to see if these individuals chose creative professions more often than the control group. Bipolars and siblings of bipolars and schizophrenics were more likely to choose a creative profession, while schizophrenics showed an increase in professions involving the visual arts. Unipolar depressives and their kin were no more likely to be involved in the creative professions than were those in the control group.

A Hungarian study led by Szaboles Keri (Keri) implicates the genotype T/T of the gene neuregulin 1 as being responsible for both psychosis and creativity in schizophrenia and bipolar. This gene is involved in neuron development and interneuron connections. The T/T form appears to enhance creativity in those of high intelligence and academic performance, possibly by decreasing prefrontal cortex cognitive inhibition.

Creativity and Hypomania

Plato defended madness as a "mantic art" (47) and believed that "madness comes from God, whereas sober sense is merely human" (47). Such an altered mood state was considered a gift from God as well as a special blessing bestowed on those who experienced it. Since the artistic temperament is universally considered to be eccentric at best and just this side of crazy at worst, the unlimited creativity, originality, inspiration, loss of inhibition, boundless energy, and free association of ideas seen in highly creative individuals can be considered a blessing and a gift. Throw in a decreased need for sleep, exaggerated self-confidence, and heightened sexuality and you have a classic description of hypomania or mild mania. Despite the advantages that hypomania or mania offers to those who have special abilities and creativity, discipline and hard work are required to see a work of art, a book, or a musical composition perfected. Original and creative ideas may arise freely during hypomania and mania but often the work of implementing those ideas is done in less elevated states of mind. Control, concentration, attention, and discipline are usually required to see big projects to the end. Dr. Sis has learned to use the ideas she has while hypomanic when she is in a more normal mood state:

> A coping mechanism, among many, is my file card system. I learned this in a "brainstorming" situation and it works to capture the brilliance while it flows, and then put it into a form that is usable later. I take a deck of colored index cards and start writing ideas as fast as I can. And that's fast when I am manic. One idea per card, or one actionable point. Flat out. Then I cut that off with my Ambien. Then, usually a week or so later, I go back and start pulling ideas from the cards. Sometimes I make categories and sort them into "do this today," "do this this week," "do this this month...." Then I methodically get something really remarkable done. So I take the brilliant moments and channel them into real projects.

Coming down from a high and even entering a slightly depressed state will help give some perspective to the work that was done while manic. Every see-saw has its balance point.

What advantage does the hypomanic state bestow on the creative individual? Studies have shown that intellectual functioning improves during hypomania, when thinking is characterized by creative and unusual solutions to problems and free association of ideas. These traits are as ideally suited for entrepreneurial endeavors as they are artistic endeavors. Abundant energy along with a decreased need for sleep and an inflated sense of self-worth enhances productivity regardless of the project, whether it's writing a book, painting a picture, composing music, or running a Fortune 500 company. Impulsivity increases, allowing for risk-taking behaviors that, if channeled into artistic or business ventures, may bring stunning successes—or disastrous failures. Ideas flow, thinking is fast and easy, and word associations are original and abundant. Kay Jamison describes hypomania as an elevated mood state where "the ideas and feelings are fast and frequent like shooting stars, and you follow them until you find better and brighter ones" (Jamison, *An Unquiet Mind* 67). The desire to spontaneously write poetry may arise due to an increase in rhyming and word associations. Puns and plays on words and witty thinking may occur. Everything is fast and easy, and it's obvious how this translates into creative writing: words are formed into phrases, sentences are crafted, and writing becomes joyful and spontaneous. Hypomanics are verbally fluent, persuasive, and supremely confident in whatever project they are involved in.

Poets have the highest rate of mood disorder and suicide among all the artistic types. Plato singled poets out for a special type of madness: "But if a man comes to the door of poetry untouched by the madness of the muses, believing that technique alone will make him a good poet, he and his sane compositions never reach perfection, but are utterly eclipsed by the performances of the inspired madman" (48). It is no wonder that the qualities of hypomania serve as the poets' muses. With heightened mood state and energy come speed of mental association, word play, and descriptive ability that might elude a slower, albeit more normal, brain. To write any literature—but especially poetry—requires using words in such a way that the reader sees and feels and experiences rather than just reads the words on the page. That's not to say poetry can't be written by normally creative folk. It can, but it can be more easily written in the heightened state of hypomania.

Like many literary artists, Virginia Woolf believed her hypomania, as well as the depression that followed, fueled the fires of her creativity. Her novels were written in a stream of consciousness style without much in the way of plot, designed to make the reader experience what the main character experiences, and her sexual ambiguity and feminist themes were ahead of their time. Such works could have come only from a mind released from the bounds of sanity: "As an experience, madness is terrific I can assure you, and not to be sniffed at; and in its lava I still find most of the things I write about. It shoots out of one everything shaped, final, not in mere driblets, as sanity does. And the six months—not three—that I lay in bed taught me a good deal about what is called oneself" (Woolf, *The Letters* 4:180).

The risk-taking, overconfidence, impulsiveness and aggressiveness of hypomania have sparked many entrepreneurial ventures, led explorers to wander the far reaches of our planet, and spurred our ancestors to leave their homelands and migrate to forge new lives in a new country. It seems obvious that people endowed with this particular set of personality traits are just the types to go out and take the world by storm. These are the movers and shakers of our society, the ones who aren't happy just sitting at home living ordinary lives. A somewhat softer set of bipolar spectrum traits classified as hyperthymia is seen in individuals who are extroverted and socially competent, enthusiastic and fun to be around, and who exude great personal warmth. These individuals are often extremely perceptive regarding the inner workings of others and may exploit this ability to either guide or control, depending on what they want to accomplish. This particular set of hyperthymic qualities are suited for leadership or entrepreneurial positions rather than for artistic endeavors, but these individuals bring their own brand of creativity to whatever they do.

Creativity and Depression

While it might seem strange to link creativity with depression—since productivity usually declines and often ceases entirely during depressed mood states—many creative bipolars feel the inspiration, ideas and experiences they have during hypomania or mild mania are reflected upon and mulled over when they are depressed, so that deeper insights achieved during their depressed state might be used later in their art or academic pursuits. When hypomanic, an individual is completely self-centered, and the truths that come to them are subjective, filtered through a haze of euphoria and feel-good chemicals that make a person's position in the world—no, the universe—important and unique. When that person is depressed, those truths are stripped of all pretense and suddenly the critical, objective personality takes over. You are nothing, you've accomplished nothing, you're worth nothing.

This stripping of all normal, adaptive delusions while depressed and seeing the world, or life, as it really is has been called "depressive realism." After all, truth is subjective and we walk around with our own delusions or versions of the truth just to get through each day. We need to believe that our lives have meaning and that we have a measure of control over what happens to us and that our choices do make a difference in how our lives turn out. If we really thought our lives were random and meaningless and our future happiness or sorrow had nothing to do with our carefully thought-out choices but were a toss of fate's dice, how could we go on? Why *would* we go on? This is the stark reality that depression forces on those who suffer from its many manifestations. It must be all the more cruel for the bipolar to be plunged from the heights of brilliance and self-importance and euphoria to the depths of despair and self-loathing.

Virginia Woolf wrote about her struggle to reconcile the hypomanic and depressed aspects of her personality as she realized that only by balancing the two Virginias could she achieve the excellence in her writing that would produce literature brilliant enough to outlive her. When she was hypomanic she could write novels but was unable or too impatient to read or concentrate long enough to write critical reviews. When she was either mildly depressed or neither depressed nor hypomanic, she could read and then write critical reviews but couldn't begin to understand how she could write a novel. Woolf was able to focus the critical "editor" aspect of her mildly depressed state on the writings of others as she wrote her critical reviews. As she became more depressed, her critical eye eventually focused on herself and her own work and life: "One goes down into the well & nothing protects one from the assault of truth" (quoted in Caramagno 70). She found her depressed mood states both frightening and exciting; her suicidal depressions frightened her, but she welcomed the stark reality and unadorned truth her depressions gave her.

The milder states of depression therefore serve as inspiration for creativity and not just as a balancing or editing function for acts of creativity produced during hypomania. That ability to become introspective, to inwardly brood about life and its meaning and one's place in the world, may actually produce beautiful poetry, music, art, or perhaps religious or philosophical insights that might not have been possible in more elevated mood states. Tchaikovsky wrote two moving and beautiful works of music during times in his life when he was depressed and recovering from manic breakdowns. His exquisite pain—as he looked back on his life with regret, yet looked at other's joy in order to find a reason to live—was poured into his music. While others might not have known the source of his inspiration, they couldn't help but feel the emotion he expressed through his music. Clearly his depression was the source of his inspiration and creativity. The Danish poet Soren Kierkegaard once said that "a poet is an unhappy being whose heart is torn by secret suffering, but whose lips are so strangely formed that when the sighs and cries escape, they sound like beautiful music" (quoted in Panter 111). Pain can be transformed into beauty by those who are willing to share their experiences, insights, and sufferings with others. Depression that becomes moderate or severe, when a person becomes nonfunctional or suicidal, is not conducive to creativity, however, and like severe mania, does not result in productivity, great insights, or works of art.

Summary

1. Creativity can be defined as the ability to respond to the world in an open and inquisitive manner and make novel connections or develop new ideas.
2. Creativity enhances whatever talents or abilities an individual has inherited, bolstered by a stimulating family environment as a child.
3. Creativity appears to be genetic in nature and is somehow linked to bipolar disease.
4. Not all creative geniuses are bipolar and not all bipolars are creative geniuses.
5. Creativity is further enhanced by the hypomanias and even the depressions of bipolar disease.
6. Non-bipolar family members also show heightened creativity, most likely representing a subthreshold or nonclinical manifestation of the disease.
7. While brilliant, creative work may be done during hypomanic mood states, refining and editing that work is often done during more normal mood states.
8. During a depressed mood state, "depressive realism," where normal adaptive delusions are stripped away and life is seen for what it is, can be a source of creative inspiration for some bipolars.
9. Enhanced creativity is possible only in hypomania, mild mania or mild depression; advanced stages of these mood states are not conducive to creativity.
10. Bipolars, and their non-bipolar family members, who possess these exceptional, creative abilities benefit from the "bipolar edge."

Chapter 14

Prominent Bipolar Disease Sufferers

Some, but not all, of the historical people listed in this chapter did not receive a diagnosis of bipolar disease while alive. The bipolar diagnosis has been inferred from historical facts and supported by a family history of mood disorder. Obviously a diagnosis made after death is based on some degree of speculation, no matter how much evidence exists to support that diagnosis. Bias will invariably be present, both in the subject's own correspondence or writings and in the writings and accounts of the subject's friends and family. Behavior must always be interpreted according to the social customs of the time and placed within historical context. This serves to prevent misinterpretation of behavior, which may be normal for a particular historical period, regardless of how abnormal it may seem to us today. Conversely, pathologic behaviors may have been socially accepted, or at least tolerated, as part of an artistic or genius lifestyle. Pathologic behaviors may also have been concealed in the historical record if considered particularly deviant and socially unacceptable, yet those very behaviors may be strong evidence for bipolar disease if viewed from a clinical perspective. Fortunately, there are usually hints of such behaviors in the historical record, often reported by close friends and family. The historical figures I've included are therefore well documented, with strong evidence of having suffered either bipolar disease or one of the bipolar spectrum disorders.

The contemporary people discussed or listed below have been open about their diagnoses and their struggle with their particular mood disorder, with only a few exceptions. In those exceptions, bipolar has been mentioned in an interview or two but was never talked about again, perhaps because of negative feedback after public disclosure. The listed individuals have exhibited classic bipolar behavior and many have a family history of mood disorder. Other names could have been added to these lists, based on behavior, but without public disclosure or reliable documentation, I cannot include them. You can find extensive lists of presumably bipolar artists, writers, musicians, and other famous, public people on the Internet; I must warn you that such lists are often poorly documented and I uncovered many mistakes as I researched each name myself. Although I did extensive research to document every person I've listed below, I have included only one source as documentation in this book, in the interest of brevity, in case you want to research a particular individual yourself.

You will notice the contemporary bipolar individuals listed in this chapter are high achievers and have been quite successful in their careers, but not all have been as successful in their private lives. While many have suffered a great deal because of their disease, mostly before diagnosis or adequate treatment, all have the benefit of modern psychiatric medication and therapy to help manage their mental illness, although not all have chosen to take full advantage of such treatment. Some of these individuals escaped diagnosis for years, with collateral damage along the way. Others either refused to take medication or were inconsistent in their medication schedule, with predictable results. The harsh truth is that the consequences of not properly managing bipolar disease can be devastating. Regardless of each individual's unique story, their bipolar successes and failures are on public view, and the courage and honestly in those who are brave enough to share their struggles with the world are commendable. The more open they are about their battle with bipolar disease, the less alone other bipolars may feel in their struggles. Perhaps you will identify with some of these people and their stories.

Some of these stories are unfortunate and a few are tragic, but I hope you will appreciate the brilliance, creativity and exceptional ability that often goes hand in hand with bipolar disease. What would the world have been like without the contributions of these incredibly talented people? The historical bipolars lived in a time when adequate medication was not available for the treatment of manic-depression, but modern histories do not have to follow the same tragic pathways of the historical bipolars. There are varying degrees of bipolar disease, as there will be in any chronic illness. Some of the individuals listed fall short of full blown bipolar-I and are instead somewhere on the bipolar spectrum, with either bipolar-II, functioning hypomania, cyclothymia, or chronic recurrent depression. Every situation is unique and delicately intertwined with an individual's basic personality as well as their particular environmental influences and underlying genetics.

Poets

Poets have the highest rate of mood disorder among the creative genius types and a listing of famous bipolar poets is impressive. William Wordsworth, a sufferer of mood swings that took the form of violent tempers, depressions, and hypochondria, penned this verse after the suicide of a young poet who suffered from the classic symptoms of manic-depression:

> By our own spirits are we deified:
> We poets in our youth begin in gladness;
> But thereof come in the end despondency and madness [Wordsworth 155].

Poets on the bipolar spectrum include William Blake, Robert Burns, George Gordon/Lord Byron, Samuel Taylor Coleridge, Emily Dickinson, T.S. Eliot, Robert Frost, John Keats, Sylvia Plath, Edgar Allan Poe, Ranier Maria Rilke, Anne Sexton, Percy Bysshe Shelley, Dylan Thomas, Walt Whitman, William Wordsworth, and William Carlos Williams, to name only a few (Jamison, *Touched with Fire* 267–68).

William Blake exhibited the classic mood swings of manic-depression with psychotic features. His admirers have always defended his "madness," including his delusions and frank hallucinations, as simply the hallmarks of a genius. Blake had a brother who, lacking William's genius, developed the reputation of being slightly mad due to his religious hallucinations (Jamison, *Touched with Fire* 66, 92–95). The Scottish poet Robert Burns, whose baseline temperament was irritable, moody, argumentative and volatile, suffered from severe and highly recurrent seasonal depressions and was prone to casual romances and sexual encounters. His parents were described as "fiery" and "subject to strong passions" (Jamison, *Touched with Fire* 67, 153). Coleridge was moody as a child and his moods worsened by the time he attended Cambridge, where his drinking, spending and whoring signaled classic manic-depressive behavior. He became addicted to opium as a way to self-medicate his agitated depressions. While Coleridge's family history isn't quite as impressive as that of some of the other poets, there is still evidence of a mood disorder in at least two close relatives, including his brother, who committed suicide at a young age (Jamison, *Touched with Fire* 67, 219–24).

Lord Byron was a classic bipolar-I with a strong family history of madness and suicide; he insisted that his depressions and other symptoms of manic-depression—his "passions" (Jamison, *Touched with Fire* 155)—were inherited from his family. Byron was extremely volatile, given to fits of violent rage, sexually promiscuity, financial overreaches, and poor judgment. His depressions were frequently agitated, consistent with a mixed mood state, and he was often suicidal and would have likely committed suicide had he not died of a fever, or its treatment, at the age of 36 (Jamison, *Touched with Fire* 69, 150–90). Byron's only legitimate child, daughter Ada Byron Lovelace, believed in "poetical science" (Toole) and was a brilliant and creative mathematician who worked with Charles Babbage on an early mechanical computer and is considered the first computer programmer. She also had the far-reaching vision of what computers could do at a time when they were being designed to do only complicated mathematic computations. Ada never had any contact with her father because her parents separated and her father left the country when she was an infant and died when she was a young child. Her mother was determined to prevent Byron's insanity in Ada by directing her intellect towards mathematics rather than poetry. But Ada exhibited the same extremes in mood and the same grandiosity, deep depressions, and some of the hypersexuality as her father; she also had a serious gambling problem. Like her father, Ada was a classic bipolar-I (Jamison, *Touched by Fire* 161–63).

Emily Dickinson suffered from such pronounced depression as a teen that she had to drop out of school, and after a panic attack at age 24 she became agoraphobic. She wrote most of the poetry in her 33-year career during an 8-year period comprised of two 4-year phases. During these phases she demonstrated heightened production in the spring and summer and decreased production in the fall and winter, signifying seasonal mood states. During the first 4-year phase, Dickinson confirmed these seasonal mood changes in letters she wrote to friends. The second 4-year phase began with an emotional upset which brought on a marked persistent increase in production in which she wrote half of the 1800 poems that comprised her body of work (McDermott). It was during this extremely productive second phase that her poetic style changed. Her symptoms during this period of increased productivity and creativity were clearly those of hypomania: "I ... cannot rule myself, and when I try to organize, my little Force explodes, and leaves me bare and charred—" (Dickinson L271). Dickinson's grandfather, the founder of Amherst College, suffered periods of depression that alternated with periods of great energy and activity.

John Keats was described as an uncontrollable child in that he was moody, volatile, nervous, and "morbid" (Jamison, *Touched with Fire* 70). He settled down somewhat and became a serious student by the age of 13 and eventually pursued medicine as a career until he realized that his medical studies prevented him from spending time writing poetry. He began to suffer depressions that he thought were caused by his conflicted feelings regarding the pull of poetry over medicine. After the publication of the first volume of his poetry, a few key people believed in Keats, despite the bad reviews the poetry had garnered. This was enough to give Keats the courage to leave medical training and pursue poetry full-time. Keats's poetry career was to be short-lived, however, as family duty took precedence as he cared for his tubercular brothers while they were dying and then, sadly, died of tuberculosis himself at age 25. Just prior to his own tuberculosis diagnosis, he began to have rapid mood swings. While there isn't enough evidence (or enough time involved, as he died so young) to diagnose classic bipolar-I, Keats may have been at least cyclothymic or bipolar-II.

Authors

Authors are an equally impressive list of sufferers: Hans Christian Anderson, Samuel Langhorne Clemens (Mark Twain), Joseph Conrad, Charles Dickens, Ralph Waldo Emerson, William Faulkner, F. Scott Fitzgerald, Graham Greene, Ernest Hemingway, Henry James, Herman Melville, Eugene O'Neill, Edgar Allan Poe (also a poet), Mary Shelley, Robert Louis Stevenson (also a poet), Leo Tolstoy, and Tennessee Williams (Jamison, *Touched with Fire* 268–69). Also Amy Tan (Eby), Patricia Cornwell (Rufus), Jack London (Goldberg 195–96), J.K. Rowling (Caruso), William Styron (Styron), and journalist and news anchor Mike Wallace (Baldoni) are bipolar or bipolar spectrum.

Ernest Hemingway's family tree is filled with bipolars, depressives, and suicides. Hemingway's physician father, Hemingway's brother and sister, and Hemingway himself all committed suicide and his granddaughter Margaux, daughter of his oldest son, committed suicide after a life-long struggle with recurrent depression, bulimia, alcoholism, dyslexia, and epilepsy. Margaux's father has no obvious evidence of a mood disorder, but another of Hemingway's sons, also a physician, is bipolar. A third son suffers from severe psychosis, presumably from a post-car accident head trauma. Hemingway's mother suffered from an unspecified nervous condition and had a nervous breakdown. The combination of mood disorders on both sides of Hemingway's parentage appears to have produced a particularly lethal combination in this family (Jamison, *Touched with Fire* 228–30).

Herman Melville's father, Allan, died of mania—bankrupt, his business in ruins. Allan's father, Thomas (Melville's grandfather), was described as eccentric, and Thomas's brother had such severe financial problems that he ended up in debtor's prison. Melville had severe mood swings, was sometimes suicidal, and would take to the sea to escape when life got too hard. One of Melville's brothers died manic, paranoid, and insane at age thirty. Another brother was plagued by debt and suffered from recurrent depression, and a paternal cousin was declared legally insane. Melville married a woman with chronic depression and their son committed suicide at age 18 (Jamison, *Touched with Fire* 216–18).

Henry James, Sr., was a tireless, restless and enthusiastic man filled with great ideas (hypomanic), and this brought him great wealth and success. Unfortunately he became an alcoholic at an early age and suffered a prolonged nervous breakdown by his early thirties. Four of his five children inherited a mood disorder. Son William James, the famous psychologist and philosopher, was depressed and suicidal as a teen. Recurrent depressions, relieved by periods of hypomania, would plaque him for the rest of his life, although they were never as debilitating as they had been in his adolescence. Son Henry James, Jr., the famous author, suffered less pronounced mood swings, although he was capable of deep depressions. Daughter Alice suffered nervous breakdowns from recurrent mixed depressions, and she was vivacious and witty (and probably hypomanic) when not depressed. William, Henry Jr., and Alice were most likely bipolar-IIs. The youngest son, Robertson, was the most severely affected, with marked mood swings and numerous nervous breakdowns; he appears to have been bipolar-I (Jamison, *Touched with Fire* 207–16).

Virginia Woolf's family history is interesting from a bipolar genetic point of view in that her mother suffered from recurrent depressions and her father was a cyclothymic, self-centered hypochondriac who had several breakdowns in middle age. All four children from this union suffered from mood disorders, ranging from cyclothymia to recurrent depressions to manic-depression/bipolar disease; a half sister was psychotic. Virginia's maternal grandfather had recurrent depressions. A paternal cousin, the poet James Stephen, was bipolar and eventually institutionalized and died of self-starvation during mania. The family was full of accomplished people, mostly writers, and Virginia's sister became a prominent artist. Virginia suffered her first breakdown at age 13 when her mother died. Her father's death when she was 22 led to a breakdown so severe she had to be institutionalized for a time. Married at age 30 to Leonard Woolf, she found great happiness both at home and in the publishing company they founded, which not only published Virginia's novels but other prominent writers' works of that day. Leonard diagnosed Virginia with manic-depression after reading some of Freud's works because he had often observed her in a state of suicidal depression, then in a state of mania he described as "violent excitement and wild euphoria" (*Beginning Again* 161) with extreme hostility and violence. Virginia's doctor believed in a biological basis for her mental troubles and recognized that families with geniuses often demonstrated periodic madness. He also recognized the connection between physical and mental stressors and the onset of symptoms, so he would prescribe a rest cure in a dark room with no stimulation with the expectation that, given time, Virginia would recover. Virginia suffered periods of mania and depression that she described as "terrific high waves, and ... infernal deep gulfs, on which I mount and toss in a few days" (*Letters* 3:237). She was extremely sensitive to what was going on around her: "I am a porous vessel afloat on sensation; a sensitive plate exposed to invisible rays" (*Moments* 133). She had visual and auditory hallucinations where she might see her long-dead mother or hear birdsongs in Greek. She attempted suicide once by throwing herself out a second-story window and again by taking an overdose of drugs.

Because of the great care that was taken to keep Virginia's daily schedule as stable, predictable, and stress-free as possible (Rose 262), she suffered only four significant breakdowns in her life. For the most part, she suffered from hypomania (Panter 236–37), which fueled her literary career and made her a spellbinding social companion. According to friend Nigel Nicolson: "One would hand her a bit of information as dull as a lump of lead. She would hand it back glittering like diamonds. I always felt on leaving her that I had drunk two glasses of an excellent champagne. She was a life enhancer" (quoted in Caramagno 49). Virginia herself commented about these hypomanic times: "Sometimes I like being Virginia, but only when I'm scattered & various & gregarious" (*Diary* 2:193). Despite the creative advantage her hypomanic state gave her, Virginia feared tipping into mania, when she would be unable to concentrate or write. She especially feared the deep, suicidal depressions because they robbed her of her self-worth, confidence, and intellect: "This is the worst time of all. It makes me suicidal. Nothing seems left to do. All seems insipid & worthless" (*Diary* 3:186). She experienced depression as a physical symptom that began with a specific type of headache or a bout of influenza rather than as a sad or depressed mood: "I am ill: yes, very likely I am destroyed, diseased, dead. Damn it!" (*Diary* 3:315). Eventually this physical manifestation of depression transitioned into a delusional, self-critical, agitated, and extremely irritable state. Virginia became convinced people were laughing at her and that she was a burden to others and especially to Leonard and she felt she should be punished. She believed her body was repulsive and the process of eating food and excreting it equally repulsive, so she refused to eat. Eventually she would take to her bed, where she resigned herself to "all the horrors of the dark cupboard of illness" (*Diary* 2:125) until her rest restored her brain into something "soft & warm & fertile again" (*Diary* 4:42) instead of "dry and parched like a withered grass" (*Diary* 4:42).

Virginia's mood swings worsened as she grew older and she began to fear that she might become permanently insane. Certain that she would never recover from the depression that was enveloping her at age 59, she wrote two suicide notes, one to her husband and another to her sister, explaining that she was hearing voices again and felt she would not recover. She wrote an additional note to her husband, a portion of which read: "Dearest, I feel certain I am going mad again. I feel I can't go through another of those terrible times. And I shan't recover this time. I begin to hear voices, and I can't concentrate. So I am doing what seems the best thing to do.... I can't fight any longer..." (quoted in Bell 226). She left the house and set out for the river near her home.

When she got there, she stuffed a large rock in her coat pocket and walked into the river until she sank and drowned.

Kaye Gibbons is a prominent native of North Carolina and a novelist who has openly talked about her bipolar disease and its influence on her writing. In numerous interviews over the years Gibbons admits she writes in hypomanic spurts that occur three or four months out of the year. Writing while hypomanic is wonderful, she says, because "you can discern those metaphors and similes very carefully and have a clear picture of the world. You seem to understand everything. Your thoughts become more eloquent and ordered and systematic. You have all the tools you need to write" (Morris). She explains that hypomanic writing is "like looking out of a very clear window and seeing the story on the other side. I have a hypersensitivity to language, and my thoughts come easily in an organized, patterned way" (Morris). While confessing that she and her doctor "play a game with the devil" (Morris) so that she remains hypomanic in order to continue writing, doing so is "like living without a net" (Morris). Once a book is finished, she is medicated down to a normal state. She called her bipolar both "a curse and a gift" (Demarr 4) but believed she was the rare bipolar who was able to "stay in charge" (Demarr 4).

Gibbons's father was an abusive alcoholic and her mother was a bipolar who committed suicide when Gibbons was 10. Gibbons was shuffled among the family, lived with a foster family for a period of time and finally, at age 13, came to live with her older brother and his wife, who provided her with a stable home and raised her. After graduation from high school, Gibbons attended college, married and gave birth to three daughters but never finished her degree. She suffered her first major depression requiring hospitalization during this time and was diagnosed as bipolar. The encouragement of a prominent Southern literature professor resulted in her producing her first novel, the prize-winning autobiographical *Ellen Foster*. Gibbons, however, could find no peace in her personal life. She was restless and changeable. Her life was full of contradictions, moves, plans, and dreams.

Sometimes she claimed she was one of the lucky ones who were able to keep their disease under control. At other times she says she never had bipolar disease in the first place, that her problems came from her dysfunctional childhood and having a creative, "odd," nature. She was at the top of her game in 2006 when someone convinced her that she was cured, and she discontinued her bipolar medications. That was the start of a downward spiral that led to her 2009 arrest for narcotics prescription forgery (Walker). The narcotics, as her lawyer stated in court, "took the edge off" her mania (Waggoner) as she struggled to complete a book she was writing at that time. She ended up with no book, no money, a narcotics addiction, criminal charges, her daughters leaving her to live with their father, and a severe ankle injury requiring the use of a wheelchair. As of 2013, Gibbons is still living with her brother and his wife. No book of hers has been published since 2006.

Musicians

The list of bipolar classical composers includes Berlioz, Beethoven, Handel, Rachmaninoff, Rossini, Schumann, Elgar and Mozart (Jamison, *Touched with Fire* 269). Nonclassical musicians and composers include Stephen Foster, Noel Coward, Irving Berlin, Cole Porter (Jamison, *Touched with Fire* 269) and Frank Sinatra (Starkey 169). More recent musicians include Hawkwind's Robert Calvert (Clerk 98), the late Kurt Cobain from Nirvana (Libby), Jack Irons from both the Red Hot Chili Peppers and Pearl Jam (Apter 134), Axl Rose from Guns N' Roses (Del James), Pete Wentz from Fall Out Boys (Schimelpfening), and Amy Winehouse (Salahi "Amy Winehouse"). Also included are Brian Wilson of the Beach Boys (Petridis), Syd Barrett of Pink Floyd ("Hungarian Research"), Ray Davies of the Kinks (Hardy), and Sinead O'Connor (Bray).

Robert Schumann was born to a probable bipolar father and a mother who suffered chronic depressions. Schumann's father had periods of extreme productivity, once writing 7 novels in an 18-month period. Multiple family members—a sister and a paternal cousin who committed suicide and two sons, one of whom became insane in his twenties and spent his life in an asylum, and the other who became a morphine addict—had symptoms of manic-depression. Schumann began to suffer dramatic mood swings by the age of 18, when he first feared he was going mad. This fear would follow him for the rest of his life. A period of hypomania occurred soon after, during which his head was so filled with music it was impossible to write down all the melodies quickly enough. This pattern of hypomania followed by deep depression would continue throughout his life. Because he was so obsessed with going insane when these hypomanic spells came upon him, he worked nearly nonstop to compose as much music as he could. In 1840, he composed over 130 songs, and in 1841 he composed an entire symphony in 4 days. Eventually his worst fear came true. At first he thought angels were singing new melodies to him. He was able to write a few of them down until he deteriorated to the point where the angels became devils that tortured him by telling him he was a sinner and threatened to throw him into hell. He hallucinated that devils were all over him like wild animals and were clawing at him. Schumann's moods violently rose and fell over the next few days until he ran out of his house and threw himself into a nearby river. After he was rescued, he was placed in an asylum, where he died two years later, at age 46, from self-starvation (Jamison, *Touched with Fire* 201–7).

Pyotr (Peter) Ilyich Tchaikovsky was born into a happy and stable family. His mother was dutiful and caring, although possibly depressed, and his father was kindly and gentle. The addition of a governess to the household found Peter begging, at age 4, to be given lessons with his older brother and cousin. It didn't take him long to pass the others in their studies, and before he was 6 years old he was reading French and German in addition to his native Russian. By the time he was 7, he was writing French poetry. Peter's musical interest seems to have been stimulated by his father's acquisition of a type of mechanical instrument that could simulate orchestral sounds via revolving cylinders, similar to a large and complicated music box. Peter showed a prodigious ability to remember complicated melodies and he began to pick them out on the piano. Fearing that he had inherited his mother's nervous condition, the governess did not encourage Peter's musical obsessions and forbid his use of the piano until the day he put his hand through a windowpane, trying to work out a melody on its surface. Only then was he allowed to use the piano and later he was allowed formal piano lessons.

Within three years, Peter had equaled his teacher in music sight-reading ability, and he not only learned musical repertoire but was able to improvise, although this often made him nervous and agitated. After spending a lively and happy musical evening at one of his parents' parties, he suddenly became very tired and went to bed earlier than usual. When the governess came up to the nursery later, she found Peter awake and weeping, pointing to his head and saying, "Oh, it's this music! Get rid of it for me! It's here, here. It won't give me any peace" (quoted in Brown 8). Peter was sent to boarding school at age 12, but he was bored and took no interest in his studies until the day his mother came to visit and took him to an opera. The experience influenced him so deeply he decided he wanted to become a composer. When he was 14, his mother died of cholera and he was devastated, but his father stepped in to watch out for him in the mother's absence. The father had always been supportive of his son's musical interests and abilities, and when he recognized Peter's growing interest in music, he insisted the school allow Peter to study music in addition to his regular schoolwork. His teachers saw no evidence of prodigious musical ability in Peter at that time, however; one later recalled that "there was nothing, absolutely nothing, that suggested a composer" (Harmon 95).

When Peter graduated he became a clerk, a job he hated but was forced to keep until he could gain entry to and study at a music conservatory. He was eventually accepted to a conservatory and began to study under some of the prominent composers of that era, but he got off to a shaky start. The coursework including conducting classes and Peter developed a delusion that his head would fall from his shoulders while he was conducting. He solved this problem by firmly grasping his chin with one hand while conducting with the other. For the rest of his life, he used this unsettling, awkward, one-handed conducting style that took orchestras by surprise until they became accustomed to it. He was also known to tear off and eat pieces of documents when he worked as a clerk, and he continued this habit during his musical career, ingesting theater programs or other excess papers. Peter's conservatory mentor harshly criticized his first orchestral score as immature (his works would always be considered unrefined) but conceded there were a few brilliant passages here and there that held promise of things to come. Over time Peter worked very hard and improved, gradually becoming more accomplished. After 10 years in an extremely productive, hypomanic state, he had built a reputation not only locally but also outside the boundaries of Russia.

Suddenly, during this productive and successful period of his life, he became restless and depressed and unable to compose. He exploded at every irritation and fought with longtime friends. Then he made the impulsive decision that he needed to marry and he did, to a girl he didn't even know who had written him a fan letter. His emotional crisis deepened and he was on the verge of collapse during the wedding, honeymoon, and early days of marriage. He attempted suicide by pneumonia by immersing himself to the waist in icy river waters one evening, hoping the extreme chill would bring on a fatal infection, but he proved to be too healthy. Eventually he collapsed into a severe mental breakdown that was considered most likely permanent. He was rescued by friends and his brother and the marriage was ended. Peter eventually recovered but relapsed when his spurned wife initiated contact again, and the irritability and paranoia returned. This time, he began to drink heavily. Much to the horror of his faithful friends and brother, Peter stole a very rare manuscript from a Venice library and wrote an inscription on the inside. Eventually he recovered and was able to reflect on those 7 months as his "brief insanity" (Brown 175). He reentered his previous hypomanic state and once again became extremely productive.

Peter's life would continue to follow this pattern of hypomanic periods of increased productivity followed by depressed periods of fatigue, irritability, social isolation, and decreased productivity. His diary entries from those years document his mercurial moods. Toward the end of Peter's life, his mood swings became more pronounced, with the depressions becoming especially severe, and he began to vocalize suicidal thoughts: "It's the devil of a life! There's not one pleasant minute—only eternal anxiety, melancholy, fear, fatigue, aversion, and so on. But now the end's already close" (quoted in Brown 427). No one knows for sure if Tchaikovsky's death at age 53 was a suicide, but it was suspicious for several reasons. It's clear that he died from cholera—the same infection that killed his mother—contracted by drinking contaminated unboiled water during a raging cholera epidemic when the water supply was unsafe. But he drank this water willingly at a restaurant, despite the protests of the staff. Peter demanded unboiled water and when it was brought to him, he grabbed the glass from the waiter before his brother could prevent him from drinking it, laughed as he knocked his brother aside, and downed the water in only a few gulps. At least one other person at the restaurant witnessed this event and was convinced that Tchaikovsky's actions were suicidal. Whether he intended to commit suicide via death by cholera, just as he attempted to commit suicide by pneumonia in the past or whether his actions were impulsive or delusional, it appears clear that he was fully aware of the risk involved in drinking potentially contaminated water. He became symptomatic by the next morning and died less than a week later.

Tchaikovsky's worsening mood swings, the lackluster critical reviews of his latest symphony performed only 9 days earlier, and his recent suicidal thoughts point strongly toward suicide as the underlying cause of his death. He had been obsessed with his Sixth Symphony (*Pathetique*) and was heartbroken at its critical failure because he had dedicated the composition to his nephew Vladimir, with whom he had a close relationship, and so had poured his heart and soul into the music. This favorite nephew would go on to commit suicide 13 years after Tchaikovsky's death. Tchaikovsky remained a tortured soul to the end:

> You see, my dear friend, I am made up of contradictions, and I have reached a very mature age without resting upon anything positive, without having calmed my restless spirit either by religion or philosophy. Undoubtedly I should have gone mad but for music. Music is indeed the most beautiful of all Heaven's gifts to humanity wandering in the darkness. Alone it calms, enlightens, and stills our souls. It is not the straw to which the drowning man clings; but a true friend, refuge, and comforter, for whose sake life is worth living" [Tchaikovsky 259].

Adam Ant was one of the most successful pop stars of the 1980s and 1990s, with a unique musical style described as British New Wave/post-punk. His unique style, costumes, and facial paint led Michael Jackson to consult him for advice regarding his own image. Adam never took his success for granted, and he approached his career from both an artistic and business perspective, creating unique music and equally creative ways to expose the public to his band to increase record sales. He didn't drink or do drugs—a rarity in the rock and roll world—and his only vice was his attraction to beautiful women. Because of his fame and looks, he could have his pick; a young Jamie Lee Curtis and Heather Graham were among his many girlfriends. Adam was born Stuart Goddard in London, England, and his mother describes him as "a horrible child with horrible ways" (Ant 7), a child who never needed much sleep and who demanded constant attention. His father was an abusive alcoholic. Living in this frightening, unstable home caused Stuart to sleepwalk and hallucinate at a very early age. These hallucinations, in which Stuart thought he was submerged in an aquarium with sea creatures swimming around him, so frightened his father that he promised to stop drinking, but he never managed to stay sober more than a couple of days. Stuart's mother finally had his father evicted when Stuart was 7 and both the sleepwalking and hallucinations stopped and life stabilized at home.

At age 21, Stuart was married and in art school while playing in a band on the side. He was living in cramped quarters with his wife at her parents' house, and for a few months after the marriage, he was happy, full of energy, and motivated to succeed. Suddenly he became dissatisfied with his life and started to obsess over music he could hear in his head that didn't sound like any music he had heard before. He felt driven to write this music down so everyone else could hear it, too. As his obsession deepened, art school was dropped, sleep came only in snatches, and he ate next to nothing. Then his hallucinations reemerged. Eventually Stuart lost his ability to concentrate or create as he spiraled downward into a severe state of depression. In an act of desperation, he grabbed a bottle of his mother-in-law's pills, swallowed a handful, and woke up in a hospital but left before they could perform electroshock therapy. He told everyone that he had killed Stuart the art student and reemerged as Adam the musician. He resumed his previous functional hypomanic state and once again felt full of creative energy as he formed a new band named Adam and the Ants. His new musical style, sparked during the hypomanic phase prior to his suicide attempt, burst on the post-punk scene and took Britain, and later America, by storm.

Adam seemed to happily exist in functional hypomania for years, driving everyone he worked with to exhaustion. Over time his untreated bipolar worsened, his life got more complicated, and his stressors began to mount. His father, who was likely bipolar, was arrested for pedophilia and eventually had a mental breakdown and became suicidal. Large sums of money began to mysteriously disappear from Adam's bank account and he became extremely stressed when he couldn't track down who was draining his funds. Inevitably his career began to wane and he slipped into depression as he lost his daily routine and a reason to get up in the morning. Adam moved to America to pursue a career in acting, but this wasn't as easy as he thought despite his fame and good looks. The change of time zones and environment both invigorated and destabilized him. A female stalker began to show up at his house in Los Angeles, so a friend loaned him a gun for protection and it soon became the focus of an auditory hallucination. He heard the gun calling to him, "Go on, load me. Squeeze the trigger and it'll be all over" (Ant 272). Adam had no idea what was wrong other than he was very depressed and fearful. Only sex seemed to soothe his angst, so he used women as a buffer between him and his illness, to keep his suicidal thinking at bay.

Finally the stressors became too much and he collapsed into what appeared to others as nervous exhaustion. He slept endlessly and when awake he shook with fear. A two-week mental hospitalization resulted in the diagnosis of bipolar disease. Adam began a period in his life where he would improve while medicated. Then he would decrease and eventually discontinue his medications once he felt stable and in control again. He recognized that he needed treatment but he didn't like the medicines' side effects so he wanted the lowest possible dose he could get by with. Sometimes he would take his medicines every other day, or only when the anxieties and fears returned, because he didn't recognize his hypomania as a part of his disease since he had been a functioning hypomanic for so long.

Eventually Adam suffered a full-blown manic attack and the feeling of being out of control truly frightened him and led to another suicide attempt. Once he stabilized, he discontinued his medications yet again while deceiving his family and friends into believing that he was complying with treatment. His mood swings became more severe, with deep, debilitating depressions requiring hospitalizations and crazy manic behaviors. One manic episode led to his arrest when he threw a car alternator through a pub window and then pointed a starter pistol at the patrons. Adam was hospitalized and the arrest and public humiliation led him to his first big breakthrough: he realized that it was the failure to take his medicine that brought on attacks, and while he was still convinced that he could manage without medication, he understood that he couldn't take that chance anymore. The first step in getting control of his life was to take his medication every single day. This caused Adam to gain weight, which was the side effect he feared the most, and the media soon began to ridicule the new, chubby Adam. He had always taken great pride in his looks because they were a big part of his public image, but he was determined to stay on treatment this time around. He hired a stylist to help choose clothing to camouflage his weight gain, but there's only so much weight you can hide.

Despite his earlier and quite sincere commitment to faithfully take his medication, Adam began to take them erratically and his mood swings returned. He got extremely manic, threatened to break in his neighbor's patio door with a shovel, then broke into a neighborhood cafe where he curled up half naked in the basement and fell asleep. He was arrested, legally sectioned (involuntarily committed) and spent six months in a hospital, where he hallucinated and then became catatonically depressed. This time he came to realize how much he wanted his life back so he could enjoy the simple comforts of his own home and spend time with his family and friends. Today, Adam understands his illness and how to manage his condition by adhering to a strict medication schedule, exercising and eating healthfully and keeping a daily routine. He understands the warning signs of trouble and knows what he can do to avoid going into a manic or depressed state. A close circle of friends and family surround Adam and support him in his daily struggles. Adam understands all too well what it's like to become a "freak show" where the ultimate taboo is "going to the madhouse" (*The Madness of Prince Charming*). Since 2010, he has been hard at work reviving his career for the sake of his daughter, who had never seen him perform. For now, at least, he appears to have his bipolar disease under control, although he was hospitalized for a month early in 2010, just as he was beginning his comeback. Since that time he has stayed stable, recorded a new album, performed in local small concert venues and successfully toured the UK, U.S., and Australia, where he was enthusiastically received. He began a second tour in August of 2013.

Artists

Artists on the bipolar spectrum include Paul Gauguin, Ernst Ludwig Kirchner, Vincent van Gogh, Michelangelo, Edvard Munch (*The Scream*), Georgia O'Keefe, Jackson Pollock, Hugo van der Goes, Francesco Bassano, Edwin Landseer, George Frederic Watts, George Innes, Pietra Testa, Henry Tilson, Mark Rothko and Dante Gabriel Rossetti (Jamison, *Touched with Fire* 269–70).

Vincent van Gogh, famous for his *Starry Night* painting, has had many diagnoses assigned long after his death to explain his various physical complaints and emotional states, including epilepsy, Meniere's disease, and even absinthe brain damage. It appears he suffered a serious mood disorder that worsened throughout his life. He had periods of delusions and psychosis and heard voices, yet had some periods of relative normalcy between his unstable times. He was unable to sustain intimate relationships, even though he very much desired to do so, as he was too moody and argumentative for anyone to want to be around him for very long. His brother, Theo, seemed to be the only one who remained faithful to Vincent, but they, too, argued at times. Vincent was a loner as a child and early on he found it difficult to get along with others. When he was 16 and working for an art dealer, he developed an adolescent crush on his landlady's daughter. This girl made it very clear to Vincent that she was not interested in him and he was hurt, as one might expect. But his reaction went well beyond teenage rejection. His appearance markedly deteriorated, he turned hyper-religious and became so rude to his coworkers and customers he was eventually fired from his job. Vincent decided to try religion as a career but failed to get into seminary, then failed to graduate from lay minister's school. When he accepted a job as a lay minister despite his lack of qualification, reports of his inappropriate behavior reached the school, which intervened, calling on Vincent's father for help in removing him from his position. Vincent gave up on religion and decided to become an artist, but he didn't last long in art school, either. He fell in love with his cousin and a repeat of his teenage experience followed. He declared his love, and his cousin rejected him; but this time he did not back down so easily. She retreated to her parents' home and when Vincent followed, they refused to allow him to see her. Vincent's response was to hold his hand in the flame of a candle until he passed out. After this incident, he lived with a woman who was most likely a prostitute, much to his parents' horror. This relationship lasted only a few months, after which he returned home to live with his parents.

Eventually Vincent moved to Paris to live with Theo and it was there that he was exposed to the works of the Impressionists. He began to use brighter colors and his artistic style changed, but he also became more argumentative and difficult to be around. It was during this period that he began to drink heavily, including large quantities of absinthe. Vincent recognized his mental and emotional deterioration and felt he needed to live in a less stressful environment, so he moved away from the city to the south of France. The move seemed to work, at least for a while. Within a few months, Vincent was clearly in a hypomanic phase, churning out two or three paintings per day. He made friends with a few of the local people although he still mostly kept to himself. Then he decided to found a school of artists—this man who couldn't get along with anyone. Theo supported the idea and even penned the solicitation letters to artists he thought might be interested. Only one artist, Paul Gauguin—another presumed bipolar—replied. Vincent developed bizarre fantasies about this artist's future role in his life. He prepared the guest room as one might prepare a room for a lover and he hoped to have many intimate walks and talks with Gauguin, each enjoying the other's company. Predictably, the two soon began to argue, as Gauguin was as emotionally labile as Vincent was. One night after an argument, Vincent cut off part of his earlobe, placed it in a box, and delivered it to a prostitute in town. Eventually Vincent was hospitalized with hallucinations and paranoia and placed in an asylum for a year. Despite his worsening mental state, the last year and a half of his life were his most productive and he created more than three hundred paintings, many of which were the best of his career. He made several suicide attempts during this period, using turpentine or paints. He initially survived his final suicide attempt, only to die from complications of the gunshot wound to his chest a day and a half later. Vincent's family was full of mood disorders, most notably his faithful younger brother, Theo, who suffered from psychotic delusions and hallucinations and could be violent at times. Another brother committed suicide. A sister suffered from lifelong psychosis and was confined to an asylum at the age of 29, where she spent the remaining 50 years of her life. Their mother suffered from chronic depression. Vincent called his and Theo's similar affliction "a fatal inheritance" (Jamison, *Touched with Fire* 234).

Science and Academia

While we usually link creativity and genius to the artistic professions, the scientific and academic professions equally benefit from innovative and original thinking and possess their share of the bipolar spectrum as well. Martin Luther was a priest who had periods of depression with such strong religious overtones he feared he would never earn his way into heaven, thus giving rise to his emphasis on faith over works in religion. During his hypomanic periods, he was extremely productive and energetic. While he may have had the clarity during his self-critical depressions to see the church for what it was at that time and to produce the "Ninety-Five Theses" he boldly nailed to the church door, it took the enormous energy of his elevated mood states to write the many theological tracts that, in clear language the common man could understand, supported his ideas, thus giving birth to Protestantism (Andreasen 85–86). Freed from priesthood and after years of a celibate life, Luther married a former nun when he was in his forties. Although he claimed he married only because his father told him to do so to carry on the family name after the death of his brothers, he found great satisfaction in his home life. He took pleasure in sex, enjoyed being surrounded by his children, and genuinely seemed to enjoy marriage, encouraging other former priests to marry just as he had done.

Yet Luther developed a severe anxious depression during this happy time in his life. He began to doubt his faith during periods of deep depression, wondering why he, of all people on earth, should have such a revelation that had ultimately led so many people away from the established church. He was tortured by the thought that if he were wrong, he had led these people to eternal damnation. His anxiety attacks brought on cardiac symptoms, sweats, and crying jags, and he was sure he was dying and damned to hell. Physically, he suffered from indigestion, constipation, hemorrhoids, and kidney stones. He treated his lack of appetite by eating voraciously, delusionally believing he was afflicted by an interior devil that could be chased away by huge quantities of food and beer as he believed the devil feared excrement. This was his excuse to gorge himself and to pepper his language with fecal references. This angry and paranoid Luther concentrated much of his fecally obsessed venom on the pope, claiming the only thing in man the pope didn't control was the rear end.

Luther was prone to vulgar, uncouth, and inappropriate topics of conversation in front of his children and guests. He teased his wife about bigamy and he belched and farted with abandon after a meal (although this may have been socially acceptable at that time). When depressed, he considered himself as excrement to be evacuated from the world's rectum. One time he had woodcuts made showing the church as a prostitute giving birth to a bunch of devils from her rectum, and he became unable to pray without also cursing, usually against the pope. He had periods of elation and excessive drinking, but he also had times when he considered himself "well," when he could see things in perspective, and was content and enjoyed life (Erikson 237–50). Even Erikson, for all his talk about childhood cleanliness training and anal obsession, describes Luther as having a manic-depressive nature (247).

Other bipolar spectrum scientists and academicians include philosopher Friedrich Nietzsche (Khazaee), physicist and mathematician Ludwig Boltzmann (O'Connor and Robertson), historian and journalist Iris Chang (Benson), philosopher Robert Corrington (Corrington), clinical psychologist and bipolar expert Kaye Redfield Jamison (Jamison, *An Unquiet Mind*), nursing pioneer and statistician Florence Nightingale ("Did Florence"), mathematician Emil Post (Urquhart 430), quantum physicist David Bohm (Peat 308–17), psychologist and author Stuart Sutherland (Sutherland), developmental biologist Lewis Wolpert (Wolpert), mathematician and author Ada Byron Lovelace (Jamison, *Touched with Fire*, 161- 63), and physicist (and inventor of the atomic bomb) Robert Oppenheimer (Matthews).

Leaders, Entrepreneurs, and Political Figures

Bipolar or bipolar spectrum leaders and political figures range from Adolph Hitler to Winston Churchill and include William Tecumseh Sherman, Abraham Lincoln, Mahatma Gandhi, Martin Luther King, Jr., Franklin D. Roosevelt, Jr. (Ghaemi 4), Christopher Columbus (Gartner 19), Oliver Cromwell, Alexander the Great, Napoleon, Lord Nelson, Alexander Hamilton, and Mussolini (quoted in Gartner 266). Other notable leaders include Democratic Missouri senator and former vice presidential candidate Thomas Eagleton (Ghaemi 258), former U.S. Representative Patrick Kennedy (Ghaemi 263), political activist Abbie Hoffman (Jezer xvii), former Illinois Democratic congressman Jesse Jackson, Jr. (Szalavitz), and Judge Sol Wachtler (Wachtler). Theodore Roosevelt, Thomas Jefferson, and John F. Kennedy appear to have had hyperthymic personalities, as do Bill Clinton and Newt Gingrich (Ghaemi 166). Wives of political leaders on the bipolar spectrum include Tipper Gore, Rosalynn Carter, Kitty Dukakis (Ghaemi 259), and Margaret Trudeau, ex-wife of former Canadian prime minister Pierre Trudeau ("Margaret Trudeau reveals"). Businessmen and entrepreneurs include publisher Philip Graham (Graham 328), Australian entrepreneur Rene Rivkin (McClymont, Connolly, and Brown), founder of Webroot Software Steven Thomas (Locke), former FBI informant and price fixer at Archer Daniels Midland, as seen in the film *The Informant!*, Mark Whitacre (Moon), and entrepreneur Ted Turner (Ghaemi 40–48).

Adolf Hitler began to experience the classic mood swings of bipolar disease in his late teens, as described by his best friend at that time. During his hypomanic periods, he became excessively talkative, restless and flighty, with the irritability and outbursts of temper of a mixed mood state. When depressed, Hitler was initially self-critical but eventually turned his criticism against the world, feeling misunderstood and unappreciated. As he left his teens behind and entered adulthood, his mood swings improved somewhat. Perhaps the discipline and regimentation of the military lifestyle served to stabilize his moodiness. Hitler's mild hypomanic traits as a young adult appear to have contributed to his leadership skills and he became quite successful in his career. The prewar Hitler was flexible and willing to listen to others, decisive and confident, capable of delegating authority, and pragmatic. He was also quite intelligent and displayed an incredible memory for detail. Yet there were early signs of what was to come. A lack of empathy in certain circumstances was evident and Hitler could sometimes be violent, killing off his rivals and sometimes his allies if they opposed him. This contrasted shockingly with his usual calm, disciplined, and self-controlled leadership style. He profited from his hypomanias, but he desired treatment for his depressions and chronic fatigue so he sought out a fashionable but questionable doctor that treated many of his friends and acquaintances. Hitler had gotten his days and nights reversed and he wanted to get back on a normal schedule. This doctor prescribed barbiturates for sleep and methamphetamine for wakefulness in the morning and for energy throughout the day. Various concoctions of male hormones and steroids along with vitamins were added to these energy shots, and eventually narcotics equivalent to OxyContin were thrown in the mix to treat various GI complaints. At first there was a shot every morning but, later, multiple shots during the day were required to keep Hitler alert and functional.

Changes in Hitler's personality predictably followed as the methamphetamine destabilized his bipolar. He became so withdrawn, paranoid, indecisive, distractible, and forgetful that those closest to him, as well as Hitler himself, began to suspect he might have neurosyphilis, despite multiple negative syphilis tests. As Hitler's obsessive-compulsive disorder worsened and he began to micromanage everything, he no longer delegated tasks or listened to advice or counsel. This mental deterioration occurred over the four years Hitler received the shots, which were the last four years of his life. He cycled harder and faster during these final years and he deteriorated so much that his top-tier generals began to ignore some of his orders. They also tried to get local psychiatrists to place him in an asylum, but those doctors were too afraid of Hitler to do so. Even his shot doctor (not a psychiatrist) changed his diagnosis from depression to manic-depression and decided to increase his shot schedule, which lessened his severe depressions (he continued to suffer from mild ones) but worsened his manias and brought on delusions.

Surprisingly, Hitler never became psychotic, although he came close. He often talked of wanting to die or of killing himself during his depressed moods, but he never actually attempted suicide until the day he knew his war defeat was imminent and he shot himself while in his bunker rather than be defeated and captured. There is at least one, and probably several, bipolar spectrum individuals in Hitler's family. His father had at least a hyperthymic personality and was described as being very energetic, but he may have been hypomanic or even manic. He was certainly hypersexual, as he was married three times and fathered children out of wedlock. Hitler's mother was his father's second cousin, so it is possible Hitler got a double dose of bipolar genes, which may have worsened his bipolar presentation. One half brother was a petty criminal, moved often, and was hypersexual like his father. Hitler's half niece, of whom he was very fond, died of a gunshot wound while living in Hitler's household. While this was declared a suicide at the time, some historians speculate that Hitler may have been romantically attached to his niece and killed her during a romantic altercation (Ghaemi 188–207).

Contrast Hitler's story to that of his contemporary Winston Churchill. While Hitler's deteriorating bipolar nearly destroyed Europe, Winston Churchill's bipolar helped save it. Churchill may have been cyclothymic, but with his pronounced and often prolonged depressions, it's more likely that he was bipolar-II. He was constantly in a state of mood fluctuation and was described by his friends and social contacts as frequently irritable and grouchy, likely representing a mixed state between his times of depression and hypomania. When hypomanic he was energetic, sociable, and impulsive, but when depressed he was plagued by suicidal thoughts and urges. Churchill could be incredibly productive when "up." He managed to write 43 books (72 volumes) and keep up with a large amount of correspondence during his lifetime. He sought treatment for his depression and was also given amphetamines, the only antidepressant known at that time, but in reasonable doses and by a reputable doctor who closely monitored him. He also self-medicated with huge amounts of alcohol. Toward the end of his life, he felt like a failure, despite his many accomplishments. This "depressive realism," while harsh when turned on oneself, allowed Churchill to recognize Hitler's danger long before anyone else in England or Europe knew what was going on. Churchill's father was hypersexual and died insane, presumably from neurosyphilis. This hypersexual behavior, a classic bipolar manic symptom, would have put him at greater risk of contracting syphilis, but the insanity could have come from bipolar psychosis as well as neurosyphilis. Churchill's daughter suffered from recurrent depressions and committed suicide, and a first cousin also suffered from recurrent depressions (Ghaemi 57–67).

Paolo Taviani, Europe's foremost authority on Christopher Columbus, calls him an "extraordinary genius" (67) whose intuition was "brilliant even in its errors" (49). Columbus believed himself to be the Messiah-like figure God had chosen to accomplish great things: "Our Lord ... opened my understanding with his hand, so that I became capable of sailing from here to the Indies and He set fire to my will to carry this out" (*The Log* xiii). This divine revelation led Columbus to embark on a mission that included a plan to recapture the Holy Land, using the gold he hoped to find in the Indies to finance a new crusade; finally, he would set the scene for the Apocalypse after he had saved all the people on earth. He changed his name to "Christoferens" (Christ-bearer) (Gartner 22) to signify his status as the man who would bear Christ across the ocean, just as legend claims Saint Christopher bore the infant Jesus across a swollen river. Thereafter he signed his name in a strange pyramidal code of letters that has yet to be deciphered. Columbus never once doubted himself: "God will cause your name to be wonderfully proclaimed throughout the world ... and give you the keys of the gates to the ocean, which are closed with strong chains" (Columbus, *The Libro* 107). He rearranged facts and events to fit his grandiose convictions, and even when events were against him his confidence that God would take care of him gave him absolute assurance that he would prevail.

When he sailed westward from the region of the Grand Canary Islands into uncharted waters, he was confident that the Indies were only a 21-day journey away and he stocked his boats accordingly. His sailors were so alarmed at these meager provisions that mutiny was an ever-present threat, as Columbus calmly reports in his log: "I am having serious trouble with the crew.... They have said that it is insane and suicidal on their part to risk their lives following the madness of a foreigner" (*The Log* 52). Miraculously, land was spotted only a week and a half past the three-week estimate, and the Bahamas were discovered. Columbus eagerly explored the area and was convinced he had found the outer islands of Japan and China. He made four voyages in all, searching in vain for the Indian and Chinese mainlands. Although he toyed with the idea that he might have actually discovered a fourth continent, he wasn't willing to fully commit to that idea, preferring instead to stick to his original belief: "Those lands which I have now discovered are at the end of the Orient" (*The Log* 190). He also believed he had discovered the entrance to the biblical

Garden of Eden off the coast of what is now Venezuela, and Solomon's gold mines, from which Solomon had built the temple in Jerusalem, in what is Panama today (Columbus, *The Voyage*).

When Columbus first conceived this holy mission, his "original and brilliant plan of reaching east by sailing west" (Taviani 42), he appealed to King John II of Portugal to sponsor his venture but was dismissed from court because his ideas were so grandiose and exaggerated that he was deemed a madman. It was obvious to the court's learned council that he had seriously underestimated the circumference of the earth and therefore the distance that would have to be sailed to reach the Indies from Europe. Contrary to what we've been taught in school about a widespread belief in a flat earth during Columbus's era, the curvature of the earth was widely accepted and was the basis for maritime navigation at that time. The earth's diameter, as well as the amount of landmass in comparison to ocean, based on the known land masses of Europe, Asia, and Africa, had been relatively accurately estimated and was used to judge Columbus's calculations of his proposed westward route to the Indies. Columbus had nothing but overblown confidence and claims of a divine mandate to back up his inaccurate calculations and ill-conceived plans. He was not deterred, however. He took his pitch to King Ferdinand and Queen Isabella of Spain and although the king soon tired of Columbus's far-fetched ideas and excused himself to go to bed, Columbus found a willing and interested audience in the queen. The two of them stayed up late that night as Columbus talked and talked and talked. It has been suggested that a sexual attraction may have drawn these two together, but it was more likely a meeting of kindred minds, both religiously fevered and inflamed by the idea of starting their own crusade. (Isabella would go on to start the Spanish Inquisition in later years.) Columbus's venture was turned over to a committee of advisors and, once again, was rejected as being unscientific and unrealistic. Following Isabella's advice, he bided his time, and four years later he appealed to the same committee and was turned down yet again. This time the denial was harsher—his plan was called "mad." The queen consoled him by promising that his project would be reconsidered with a different committee sometime in the future. In 1492, nearly 15 years since his first meeting with Queen Isabella, she sent for Columbus and convened a new committee of academics to consider the venture and this time the vote was split. Isabella cast the deciding vote in Columbus's favor and suddenly his long-awaited plan became a reality.

Immediately, in an outrageous display of grandiosity, Columbus began to make demands that stunned the court. Not only did he demand titles that only the royal family held, he also wanted full control of all lands he discovered and 10 percent of all profits. He became enraged at any attempts on the part of the royal couple to negotiate, so he was denied everything. Spain's minister of finance eventually intervened and explained to the royal couple that as outrageous as Columbus's demands were, if he were to deliver the goods, 90 percent wasn't a bad profit and it was certainly better than nothing, which was exactly what they would get if Columbus didn't at least try. He pointed out that if Spain didn't find the sailing route west to the Indies, some other European nation eventually would if it were possible; and if there were riches to be had, Spain had better be first in line to get them. The king and queen reversed their decision and agreed to all of Columbus's demands. They gave him his titles (Knight, Don, High Admiral of the Ocean Sea, Viceroy and Perpetual Governor) and the control he wanted. Then they waited, hoping it would pay off in the long run. In the end, Columbus made some money and his titles elevated his societal status, but he never found the huge piles of gold he was so sure were waiting for him at the end of his delusional rainbow. And while he never saw his holy crusade materialize or came close to fulfilling his God-given mandates, he made a discovery that altered the history of the world, although he remained delusional about his discovery until his death. Columbus was hypomanic, driven, and grandiose in the beginning, but he became increasingly delusional, probably manic, and possibly psychotic as time progressed.

He compiled a collection of biblical and religious prophecies that he called *The Book of Prophecies,* proving, in his opinion, that he was the one person on earth chosen by God to fulfill them. One of his biographers, Gianni Granzotto, used this prophesy book as proof that Columbus finally broke from reality and became mad (Gartner 24). Intense religious experiences, divine revelations and prophesies, and religious ecstasies are not uncommon in hypomania and mania. There is little fundamental difference between religious fervor and entrepreneurial zeal—the qualities that ignite one feed the other—and Columbus exhibited both traits. He may have been on a mission from God, but he drove a hard bargain in order to elevate his social status and lay aside riches in this world, despite his claims that he would use those riches to fund a new crusade. Columbus had an unshakable belief in himself, despite the fact that the experts and academics of the day, and even his own crew of seasoned sailors, believed his plan was impossible. Big ideas, big egos, and big goals—all hypomanic traits—sometimes make for big discoveries, big business ventures, and world-changing events. Columbus accomplished all three.

He is called the "Mouth of the South" because he speaks his mind and often makes outrageous statements. His hypomania and grandiosity are obvious in statements such as this one: "I went 90 miles an hour through my career. I built a multibillion-dollar company, and I won the America's Cup. I was the greatest sailor in the world. I ran through three wives and numerous girlfriends, and I wore them all out! I smoked through life! I'm still going fast!" (Sellers). Ted had mood swings as a child but claims they were a result of his being sent away to a boarding school for a couple of years when he was 4 while his father was in military service. He suffered from anxiety which he blamed on his unstable and often difficult childhood; he was singled out by his alcoholic, stern father for mean, often abusive discipline. Ted's aunt describes the father's brutal behavior as "almost like a Dr. Jekyll and Mr. Hyde" (Turner 7) and recalls a time when a doctor making a house call found suspicious bruises on young Ted's body. By the time Ted was 10 he had become less moody, but he feels this was a conscious decision he made in order to develop a more positive attitude toward his life. Describing himself as a "restless kid" (4) who did mischievous but not mean things, Ted was kicked out of the private school he attended for first grade and entered public school, where, he says, his behavior was unchanged but tolerated. He says he'd most likely be diagnosed as having attention deficit disorder today, but he believes his behavior was the result of being alone in the boarding school for so long and craving attention at whatever the cost. Ted stayed in public school until the fifth grade, when his father decided to send him to a military boarding school. He then brought Ted home for the sixth grade, then sent him back to a different military boarding school in the seventh grade. At first Ted got into trouble and was determined to be the worst cadet possible short of being expelled, but by the time he was a junior he had done a complete turn around and decided to be the best cadet at the school. He distinguished himself on the debate team, leading the school to its first state championship in 30 years, largely due to his creative interpretation of debate topics.

Ted's father, Ed, had a severe mood disorder and was most likely bipolar-I. Ted describes him as a complicated man—moody, volatile, quick tempered, unpredictable, a philanderer, and a perfectionist, but also a deep thinker, charming, and brilliant at business. He made Ted work summer vacations starting when he was eight years old. By the time Ted was 12, he was working a full workweek during the summer with the crews that did the toughest outdoor jobs at his father's company. Even though Ted extracted a promise from his father that he would commit to pay for four years of college, his father suddenly withdrew all financial support at the start of Ted's junior year when he became displeased with Ted's choice of a nonbusiness major, despite the fact that the college did not offer a business major. Ted loved the family business, so after a brief time of rebellion once he was forced to leave college, he settled back in at home and found his place in lower management and began to work his way up. He watched his father expand the company and orchestrate a merger that put the company in significant debt that would hopefully pay huge dividends in the future. Ed, however, began to fall apart, triggered in part by the stress of the huge financial debt the company now shouldered. Ted had a front row seat to this breakdown but didn't know what to do about it. Describing his father as manic after a time when his mood swings had become more pro-

nounced, Ted recalls: "Dad was elated—the most energized I'd ever seen him....
[T]his upbeat behavior came just as he was approaching the brink of a collapse.
He was like an engine that runs at its fastest right before stripping its gears"
(55). Suicide followed not long after, and Ted was left to run the company,
which, under his leadership, went from a successful local business to a billion-
dollar enterprise. Ted was diagnosed with bipolar late in life (those around
him describe at least a volatile, cyclothymic temperament at that point,
although he was probably a functioning hypomanic for many years). He was
treated with lithium for a time but claimed it did nothing for him, although
his ex-wife Janie, the woman he left Janie for, and Jane Fonda have all claimed
otherwise (Ghaemi 44). In fact, his girlfriend at that time said that "with
lithium he became very even tempered. Ted's just one of those miracle cases
... lithium is a miracle" (Painton).

A different psychiatrist some years later dropped the bipolar diagnosis
and instead "diagnosed" Ted with high motivation and drive, episodes of anxiety, and no depression, and Ted terminated his lithium treatment. At that time,
bipolar spectrum disorders generally weren't recognized, so if an individual
wasn't classically bipolar-I they weren't likely to get diagnosed. Ted most likely
wasn't the best historian, particularly since he'd been on lithium for some years
and may have forgotten what he had been like before treatment, or perhaps he
never had any insight into his hypomanic or manic behavior in the first place.
Jane Fonda, Ted's third wife, has said that "he needs constant companionship
and keeping up with him can be exhausting. It's not just all the constant activity—it's his nervous energy that almost crackles in the air.... He has to keep
moving" (quoted in Turner 329). Teddy Turner, Ted's oldest son, remembers
that time with his father during childhood was spent at a "frantic pace" having
"maximum fun" (quoted in Turner 77). Ted is not bipolar-I like his father was.
But with his family history and his restless, nervous energy, creative thinking,
extreme confidence, risk taking in business ventures, volatility, and his habit of
living full throttle, he is assuredly somewhere on the bipolar spectrum. As a
young man, Ted reported that he often drove 120 miles per hour and was once
nearly hit by a train while whizzing across railroad tracks (Ghaemi 41).

When I was living in the South Carolina low country, not far from Ted's
home where his second wife and children lived and where he spent weekends
when he was working in Atlanta, I experienced his manic driving myself as I
traveled on a country back road on my way to my Saturday moonlighting job.
I saw an expensive car going at least 90 mph down the center highway line
toward me. Boys in baseball uniforms had their arms and heads out the windows, banging on the sides of the car, obviously celebrating an early-morning
ballgame win. A head-on collision was inevitable unless I drove my car off the
road and wrecked, as I assumed the driver was distracted and had no idea I

was on the road in front of him. At the very last minute the car swerved into its own lane and blew past me. When I got to the hospital for work, I asked if anyone had any idea who would be recklessly driving an expensive car full of kids on that particular back road. "Oh, yes, that must have been Ted Turner heading back to his place," I was told. "He always drives like that."

Hypomanic traits have obviously contributed to Turner's entrepreneurial successes and made him a billionaire. He was incredibly creative in the way he approached business and was willing to take huge risks in hopes of future gain. Turner was able to look at things from a different angle than everyone else, recognize opportunities where others didn't, then had the guts to take chances that others were too afraid to take. Interestingly, Turner seems to be more realistic than the average entrepreneur, which may be the secret to his string of successes: his risks are generally carefully calculated. Even more interesting, his biggest failure—the Time Warner merger—came in the years after he was taken off lithium. This first real failure was truly a spectacular one. He lost 80 percent of his fortune. Not only did Ted's hypomanic traits make him an excellent entrepreneur but they also helped him be resilient to failure: "I lost Jane. I lost my job here [CNN]. I lost my fortune, most of it. I have a billion or two left, you can get by on that if you economize. But I was worth seven or eight billion at one point. But I—you carry on. And I found other things to do" (Kurtz).

Actors

We would expect a high number of bipolar individuals in the highly creative field of entertainment: actors Ned Beatty (Purse, "Ned Beatty"), Catherine Zeta Jones (Salahi, "Catherine Zeta-Jones"), Marilyn Monroe (Oliver), Patty Duke (Duke), Russell Brand (Brand), singer and actress (and George Clooney's aunt) Rosemary Clooney (Clooney 213–22), Richard Dreyfuss (Smith), Stephen Fry (Gallagher), Vivien Leigh (Holden 183), Jim Carrey (Leung), Drew Carey (Stossel and Sullivan), Carrie Fisher (Fisher), Hugh Laurie (Dos Santos), Linda Hamilton ("Linda Hamilton says"), Jean-Claude Van Damme (Purse, "Jean-Claude Van Damme"), Owen Wilson (Kliff), and Winona Ryder (Goodwin). Dick Cavett and Marriette Hartley ("Larry King"), Jane Pauley (Pauley), Mel Gibson (Murray and Maddox), Spalding Gray (Williams), Margaux Hemingway (Landau), Jenifer Lewis ("Actress Jenifer Lewis"), Kristy McNichol ("Kristy McNichol"), Burgess Meredith (Tank), *Upstairs, Downstairs* actress Nicola Pagett (Pagett), and Jonathan Winters (Dowell) are bipolar or on the bipolar spectrum.

Carrie Fisher has been open about her bipolar disease and the addictive self-medicating behaviors that go along with it, going public in 2000 once she recovered from an acute psychotic episode and psychiatric hospitalization in 1997. In February of 2013, she had a very public acute manic episode when she was the celebrity entertainment onboard a cruise ship. This episode resulted in a second, albeit brief, psychiatric hospitalization. Although she has no memory of the episode, video taken by audience members shows her slurring her words and rambling while her dog urinates and defecates onstage, Fisher apparently oblivious to what is going on. She says she wasn't psychotic but severely manic and extremely delusional, believing everything she looked at had meaning or was a sign or warning. She couldn't sleep, was agitated, and felt tremendous pressure to write: "I was writing on everything. I was writing in books. I would have written on walls" (Leonard).

Carrie grew up in Hollywood where "normal" is bipolar by definition, so she thought her nonstop talking, sleepless nights, drug addictions and rehab stints were par for the course. A bipolar diagnosis at 24 didn't phase her. She continued with her own cocktail of illegal and prescription drugs, washed down with alcohol, and haphazardly took her bipolar meds when it suited her. Predictably, her mood swings and nonstop talking worsened over time. She suffered two failed marriages but produced a daughter from her second marriage. Eventually she stopped all her bipolar meds, not that she had ever been all that faithful in taking them. Her increasing high manias, her worsening depressions, and her addictions began taking a toll on her relationship with her daughter. Carrie knew she needed help but she couldn't bring herself to take the first step. It took six manic days and the sleepless nights that followed, as well as the acute psychotic episode that manic week, to get Carrie's attention. She thought the television was talking about her and to her; she was all the characters on the news show she was watching. Her brother had her committed and when she was asked to sign her name on the commitment papers, she signed "Shame." Carrie uses humor and a razor sharp wit to deal with her bipolar. She says she has waited her entire life to get an award for something. She knows it won't be for her acting and had hoped it would be for her writing. But at least she gets awards all the time for being mentally ill, which she jokingly says she must be good at: "How tragic would it be to be runner-up for Bipolar Woman of the Year?" (Fisher 131).

Athletes

Athletes are also well represented in the bipolar spectrum, but the attitude in sports toward mental "weakness" is not conducive to full disclosure of any type of mental illness. You will notice in the list below that non–American athletes appear to be more willing to disclose their diagnosis. Slowly but surely, the stigma has begun to wane somewhat and a few athletes are beginning to speak up, but mostly as an explanation for out of control or inappropriate behavior: Mike Tyson (Jenkins), British boxer Frank Bruno (Brockes), English footballer Paul Gascoigne ("Paul Gascoigne: What Gazza Did"), Australian footballer Jonathan Hay (Horan), Australian rugby player Andrew Johns (Weaver), Scottish racing cyclist "The Flying Scotsman" Graeme Obree (Roe), former Oakland Raiders NFL pro Barret Robbins ("Agent: Robbins"), cricket player Michael Slater ("Slater reveals"), rugby player Tim Smith ("Tim Smith leaving"), NBA basketball player Delonte West (Berger), baseball player Darryl Strawberry (Borden) and former NFL football player Dimitrius Underwood (Sallie James).

Paul Gascoigne, or Gazza as he is called, was once considered the most talented British footballer to have ever lived; but his stunning sports career derailed in a mess of domestic violence, clown suits, bulimia, compulsive gambling, obsessive-compulsive disorder, and, most spectacularly, alcoholism (Gascoigne, *My Story* and *Being Gazza*). He first had suicidal thoughts at age 7, developed twitches and obsessions at age 10, for which he received therapy for a short time before his father terminated the sessions, and then began to suffer depressions at age 13. He developed a gambling addiction (gaming machines) in his teens and shoplifted to get gambling money (Stewart). For a time sports seemed to calm his demons, but eventually his life continued its downward spiral. He was involved in a drunk-driving accident early in his career and at first claimed that his car had been stolen before finally admitting guilt. He was constantly in trouble with his team managers for misbehavior, but he felt he was being picked on. Once he attempted to drive a tractor into the dressing room to show his displeasure at being disciplined, jumping off just before it hit the building. Later in his career, his behavior on and off the field became more and more outrageous and unsportsmanlike until he was finally dropped from his team. His response was to fly into a rage and attempt to destroy his team manager's office. He never played football in England again after that incident. His career was over.

The first time Gazza had any real therapy was when he was hospitalized after drinking 32 shots of whisky in one sitting. His manager at the time admitted him to the hospital while Gazza was unconscious and unable to object, but he only stayed half of the recommended 28-day hospitalization. Several years later, he was sent to America for treatment at a clinic in Arizona, where he would go two more times in the next few years after relapses. It was at his initial clinic visit that he received his bipolar diagnosis. After he suffered a spine injury while training for a TV show, Gazza got addicted to opioid pain killers, which set off a predictable chain reaction. His obsessive-compulsive disorder worsened, he began to drink again, and he became addicted to Red Bulls, drinking up to 15 cans a day. A year later, he developed pneumonia and while sick got his drinking under control, but his sobriety didn't last long. Several years later, he was committed under the Mental Health Act for bizarre behavior while staying in a hotel in northern England. Since that time, Gazza has been plagued by legal problems, drunk-driving incidents, and cocaine possession. He appeared at the scene of a police stand-off with a murderer, claiming to be his friend and insisting he had brought him a "can of lager, some chicken, a mobile phone and something to keep warm" (Collins). In February 2013, Gazza was back in Arizona, undergoing rehab again. His alcohol withdrawal was so severe he was placed in an intensive care unit for a time ("Paul Gascoigne in Intensive Care"). He relapsed by June 2013 and had one hospitalization and more arrests for drunkenness and assault up to August 2013.

Summary

1. The individuals in this chapter have made enormous contributions to society, despite considerable challenges and, all too often, suffering and sometimes tragedy.
2. Some of these individuals have singlehandedly changed the course of history.
3. Most parents would not deliberately choose to pass down the more severe manifestations of the bipolar spectrum to their children.
4. The creativity, energy and genius in many of these bipolar individuals are highly desirable traits in our society.
5. What would happen if the ability to diagnose the susceptibility to bipolar disease were to be discovered in the future and parents will be given the option to abort "afflicted" fetuses?
6. In the above scenario, would our society lose our future Schumanns, Van Goghs, Emily Dickinsons, Lord Byrons, Ted Turners, Winston Churchills, and Martin Luthers in order to prevent a Hitler from being born?
7. Would our history be forever altered with the loss of these creative souls whose minds soar past the bounds of society's constraints in ways that less creative brains can't begin to fathom?
8. The answer is yes, our world would be forever altered without the contributions of these brilliant bipolars.
9. Our world always has been and always will be a better place because bipolars live among us.
10. We must continue to find ways to ease the suffering and prevent the tragedies the disease often carries with it while allowing its special gifts to thrive.

Chapter 15

Putting It All Together

Recovery is the process of seeking mental wellness in the context of experiencing bipolar disorder.

—Mountain 108

This book has attempted to educate you about all aspects of bipolar disease. I hope you know more now than when you first began to read it. Now it is up to you to put what you have learned into practice. Getting your diagnosis, learning about bipolar, and then getting your disease under good medical control is only the start in learning to live your life successfully with bipolar disease. Keeping ahead of your disease will require daily effort, but the harder you work to get control the easier it will be to stay in control.

Get Control and Keep Control

Despite the best drugs and the most vigilant adherence to dosing schedules, life happens. Many things occur that can disrupt a bipolar's body rhythm and cause a little crack in the dike that may ultimately threaten stability if the disruption continues. You can't just rely on your medications. You must be vigilant on a daily basis for all the ways life can trip you up, and then you must be ready to fix what went wrong, no matter how small or insignificant it might seem, because even little things add up over time. You'll learn what your thresholds are—whether losing two nights of sleep will bring on a mood swing or whether it takes a month of poor sleep to do that. Fair or unfair, some bipolars will have to be more rigid in their daily routines than others in order to gain control over their disease. Other bipolars may be able to live fairly normal lives with just a watchful eye toward impending trouble. Everyone is different and you will soon learn what your limits are.

The more people you have on your team, watching for signs of disease in the future, the better. There's always the problem of paranoia as the disease begins to creep up on you, so choose your support team wisely and remind yourself that even if you feel distrustful and paranoid toward them, you have personally chosen these people and they have your best interests at heart. Even Mrs. Mamone became frustrated when her family didn't believe her psychotic hallucinations, but she trusted them enough to agree to come in for a psychiatric assessment and the hospitalization that resulted from her evaluation. Research has found that bipolars with social connections do better than those who are loners, as long as those social connections are positive and healthy and nonstressful.

Relationships with family and friends may be strained at times, as bipolars tend to be egocentric and expect a lot from their friends and family and have intense feelings regarding their relationships. This may ignite intense arguments at times, even when only mild symptoms are present. To live in this world, to work, to play, and to thrive, you have to interact with people. Unless you decide to live as a hermit, you have to work, buy groceries, pump gas, get your hair cut, go to the post office, and speak to your neighbor. You need people and people need you. It's to everyone's benefit that you learn to have healthy relationships and that you nurture them along the way. You do not want to wear out your friends, family or coworkers by being overly intense, needy, or possessive. I guarantee that your friends and family give to you much more than you give to them, even if you don't believe that's true. Learn to give back in healthy ways.

The Goal: Remission

Regardless of the chronic illness, true cure is almost never possible. Remission is what you work for and hope for and enjoy once it's achieved. Attacks will occur. But with hard work, you hope to limit your attacks so they remain mild and infrequent. It is tempting, when remission is prolonged, to believe you are cured. A missed medication dose here and there may stretch into days, then weeks, then months. A disruption in your schedule now and then may slowly become a habit, until your carefully crafted stable lifestyle is gone. The careful monitoring of your moods or life stressors might be dropped because you don't seem to need those things anymore. You might drop out of talk therapy or your support group and thereby lose an objective opinion regarding emerging symptoms. This is when bipolar disease creeps up on you. You aren't paying attention, so you don't notice the disease is coming back. But those around you most likely do. Or maybe you do notice but you don't want to admit that it's coming back when you thought it was gone forever. The longer you ignore what's going on, the harder it's going to be to regain control.

You can never let down your guard when you are in remission. Taking your medications, living a stable lifestyle, participating in some form of talk therapy, and having the support of friends and family are what helped you achieve remission in the first place. The more you tinker with this formula, the more likely you are to come out of remission. The key to successfully managing your bipolar is to know about bipolar disease in general, then know how bipolar disease is expressed in you. You may not always be aware of how your symptoms appear to others, so you need friends and family to give you this information. You need to lower your risk of having a mood episode, which means watching out for life stressors, not abusing drugs or alcohol, getting enough sleep, trying to keep interpersonal conflicts to a minimum, and faithfully taking your medications. You also need to monitor your stress level and your moods. Keep a good, healthy daily routine; have some form of talk therapy, and maintain strong relationships with friends and family. Your mental health professional will guide you to the right medication, the right therapy, and the right lifestyle management plan. This is a tall order, but remission, or "recovery," from bipolar disease is well worth the effort.

Acceptance

Realistically, not everyone is going to achieve the same level of remission. Some individuals will retain a great deal of symptomatology and struggle to prevent relapse, while others will remain relatively normal and have only infrequent relapses. It is up to you to determine how stable or sensitive you are to triggers and stressors and then do what you need to do to stay healthy. As Hornbacher says, "This isn't the end of the world. It's just the way things are. Managing mental illness is mostly about acceptance—of the things you can't do, and the things you must" (277). Many bipolars struggle with acceptance because they don't want to give up their hypomanias, although they never want to experience another severe depression again. But you can't have it both ways. To stabilize your moods, your hypomanias and manias must be controlled as much as possible in order for you to prevent your depressions. After years of going off and on lithium because she was ambivalent about treatment, Jamison finally realized that her enjoyable manias were becoming mixed and suicide was becoming more of a threat as her depressions worsened: "I miss the lost intensities, and I find myself unconsciously reaching out for them ...These current longings are, for the most part, only longings, and I do not feel compelled to re-create the intensities: the consequences are too awful, too final, and too damaging" (*An Unquiet Mind* 212).

Jamison goes on to say this: "I have often asked myself whether, given the choice, I would choose to have manic-depressive illness. If lithium were not available to me, or didn't work for me, the answer would be a simple no—and it would be an answer laced with terror" (*An Unquiet Mind* 217). Many bipolars, when asked if they would choose a life without bipolar, say they wouldn't give up the heightened experiences they've had during their hypomanic or manic times or even the lessons they've learned during their depressed times, as Jamison explains:

> So why would I want to have anything to do with this illness? Because I honestly believe that as a result of it I have felt more things, more deeply; had more experiences, more intensely; loved more, and been more loved; laughed more often for having cried more often; appreciated more the springs, for all the winters; worn death "as close as dungarees," appreciated it—and life—more; seen the finest and the most terrible in people, and slowly learned the values of caring, loyalty and seeing things through [218].

This doesn't necessarily mean Jamison and other bipolars crave those experiences anymore, but they have learned to accept them as part of their life and have come to terms with the good and the bad experiences of their disease in order to move forward in recovery. This is what all people with a chronic illness have to do in order to live a relatively normal life that isn't completely defined by their disease.

Hornbacher's first book, *Wasted*, which was nominated for a Pulitzer Prize, chronicled her teenage struggle with an eating disorder before she was diagnosed with bipolar as an adult. She is a gifted writer who was amazingly successful despite a chaotic, psychotic, drunken, and often suicidal lifestyle. When asked if she missed anything about her life before she got her bipolar under control, she explained how stability is better than her previous manic highs:

> People ask me this often, and I honestly have to say that the answer is no. The exhilaration of the old manias, which we all love for a while and in a way, was always accompanied by that horrific crash, which got worse and worse over time. So these days, instead of manic exhilaration, I have the wonderful experience of genuine happiness, joy, excitement—all those feelings that I chased when I chased mania before, because I thought mania was the only way I could get those feelings. Turns out I was wrong. A healthy, stable life brings me far more joy and excitement than mania ever did. Also, I truly believed my creativity stemmed from the illness, and I could only reach creative generation in an altered state of mind. Wrong there too. I produce vastly more, and vastly better, work when I'm healthy, because I have the stability to work consistently, and consistently strive to improve ["Interview"].

If you think that a normal, stable life isn't worth working for, or is too much trouble, you need to read Jamison's book, and Hornbacher's and Behrman's and Cheney's and Vonnegut's. All of them have severe bipolar-I disease, and it's a miracle they are alive today. Yet each enjoys a stable, normal life in ways you might not be able to imagine now. You owe it to yourself to do whatever you can so you, too, can experience stability for yourself.

The End—and the Beginning

Robert Corrington is a philosopher who battled bipolar for many years before he was diagnosed (despite having a mother and sister with the disease), and he suffered consequences in his personal and professional life although the brilliance and creative thinking that came with his bipolar also enhanced his career. This is what he has to say to other sufferers of the disease, in his book, *Riding the Windhorse*:

> Finally, I want to say a word directly to those of you who know the demons and angels of manic-depressive disorder in a deeply personal way. I have seen lives ruined and I have seen lives transfigured by manic-depression. With you I have experienced those blinding moments of sheer lucidity in which the world seemed to open up its deepest and most closely regarded secrets. And with you I have experienced those moments when time froze in its tracks and the world turned to gray on gray and all meaning drained away into a psychic black hole. With you I have considered suicide, and with you I have felt like a god incarnate.
> And with many of you I live in mourning for a self taken away by medication, a self that still beckons to me even though I know I cannot bring it back. And, in the end, with you I have struggled to find wholeness that will not be eroded by the winds of this disease [ix–x].

Corrington spend most of his life not understanding what was wrong with him, but once he did he worked hard to get his bipolar under control. You have your diagnosis and you have the information, so what are you going to do now? You can choose to let the disease control you or you can control the disease. The choice is yours. I'll let Carrie Fisher have the final say on what it takes to handle this disease, day in and day out:

> In my opinion, living with manic depression takes a tremendous amount of balls. Not unlike a tour of duty in Afghanistan (although the bombs and bullets, in this case, come from inside). At times, being bipolar can be an all-consuming challenge, requiring a lot of stamina and even more courage, so if you're living with this illness and functioning at all, it's something to be proud of, not ashamed of. They should issue medals along with the steady stream of medications one has to ingest [159].

Resources

- ACTA (Assertive Community Treatment Association)
  http://www.actassociation.org/
- Active Minds on Campus
  A college/university mental health advocacy group
  http://www.activeminds.org/
- American Association for Marriage and Family Therapy
  www.therapistlocator.net/index.asp
- American Psychological Association
  locator.apa.org
- Behavioral Cognitive Therapy
  www.abct.org
  www.beckinstitute.org
- Bipolar PDF
  http://www.nimh.nih.gov/health/publications/bipolar-disorder/index.shtml
- Bipolar Significant Others
  For friends and family of the bipolar
  http://www.bpso.org/
- Bipolar World
  Informational, ask-a-doctor link
  http://www.bipolarworld.net/
- Child and Adolescent Bipolar Foundation 1000 Skokie Blvd, Suite 570 Wilmette, IL
  60091 Phone: (847) 256–8525 E-mail: cabf@bpkids.org
  www.bpkids.org
- Depression and Bipolar Support Alliance (DBSA) 730 North Franklin St, Suite 501
  Chicago, IL 60610–7224 Phone: (312) 642–0049 (local) or (800) 826–3632 (toll-
  free); Fax: (312) 642–7243
  http://www.dbsalliance.org
- Depression and Related Affective Disorders Association (DRADA) 2330 West Joppa
  Rd, Suite 100 Lutherville, MD 21093 Phone: (410) 583–2919 E-mail: drada@jhmi.edu
- Harbor of Refuge Organization
  Peer to peer support
  http://www.harbor-of-refuge.org/
- Illness Management and Recovery Program (IMR)/SAMHSA
  P.O. Box 42557
  Washington, DC 20015
  Mon.–Fri. 8:30 A.M.–12:00 a.m. EST
  Phone: (800) 789–2647

http://store.samhsa.gov/product/Illness-Management-and-Recovery-Evidence-Based-
Practices- EBP-KIT/SMA09–4463
• International Foundation for Research and Education on Depression (iFred) 2017-D
  Renard Court Annapolis, MD 21401 Phone: (401) 268–0044 Fax: (443) 782–0739
  E-mail: info@ifred.org
• Internet Mental Health
  Informational, downloadable mood charts, information on new medications
  http://www.mentalhealth.com/
• Interpersonal and Social Rhythm Therapy (IPSRT)
  http://www.ipsrt.org/
• Medline Plus Bipolar Information
  NIH publications and clinical trials
  http://www.nlm.nih.gov/medlineplus/bipolardisorder.html
• Mental Health America
  2000 North Beauregard St., 6th Floor
  Alexandra, VA 22311
  Phone: 703–684–7722 or 800–969–6642
  Fax: (703) 684–7722
• Mental Health Recovery and Wellness Recovery Action Planning (WRAP)
  www.mentalhealthrecovery.com
• MentalHelp.net
  Information in advances in mental health
  http://www.mentalhelp.net/
• NAMI ACT Web site: http://www.nami.org/Template.cfm?Section=ACT-TA_Center
• National Alliance on Mental Illness (NAMI) Colonial Place Three 2107 Wilson Blvd,
  Suite 300 Arlington, VA 22201–3042
  www.nami.org Phone: (703) 524–7600 (local) or (800) 950-NAMI (6264) (toll-free);
  Fax: (703) 524–9094
• National Institute of Mental Health. Bipolar Fact Sheet http://www.bipolarworld.net/
  pdf/NIMHbipolarresfact.pdf
• National Institute of Mental Health (NIMH) Public Information and Communications
  Branch 6001 Executive Blvd, Rm 8184, MSC 9663 Bethesda, MD 20892–9663 Phone:
  (301) 443–4513 (local) or (866) 615–6464 (toll-free); Fax: (301) 443–4279 Fax Back
  System, Mental Health FAX4U: (301) 443–5158 E-mail: nimhinfo@nih.gov
• Pendulum Resources
  Research and medical sources
  http://www.pendulum.org/
• PsychCentral.com
  Information, extensive blog list, chat sessions
  http://psychcentral.com/
• Personal Websites and Blogs
  http://bipolarhappens.com/bhblog/
  http://blogs.philadelphiaweekly.com/trouble/
  http://blogs.psychcentral.com/bipolar/
  http://enduringbipolar.blogspot.com/
  http://kansassunflower.blogspot.com/
  http://mental-health-issues-madison.blogspot.com/
  http://mycrazybipolarlife.wordpress.com/
  http://natashatracy.com/
  http://suddenlybipolar.wordpress.com/
  http://www.bphope.com/bphopeblog/
  http://www.electroboy.com

http://www.havingbipolar.com/
http://www.healthline.com/health-blogs/bipolar-bites
http://www.healthyplace.com/blogs/breakingbipolar/
http://www.manicmoment.org/
http://www.mcmanweb.com/
http://www.time-to-change.org.uk/category/blog/bipolar

Movies, Documentaries, Videos

Adam Ant: The Madness of Prince Charming: BBC Documentary, 2004. Not available in the U.S. but can be seen in 8 parts via YouTube.

While Adam fans may be disturbed to see their beautiful boy-toy idol a middle-aged, jowly man, his inner beauty shines through in his honesty in sharing his struggles with bipolar disease. Included in this documentary are comments from former band members who struggled to keep up with Adam's hypomanic pace during the band's heyday. My only criticism of this documentary is that it is too short. I was left wanting to know more about Adam's ongoing struggle with mental illness.

Bipolar: A Manic Depressive Illness. Documentary, YouTube.

If you don't have the time to watch *up/down* (see below) this similar, excellent documentary of half the time features six bipolars discussing various aspects of living with and managing their bipolar disease. The director of the Mood Disorders Unit at Prince of Wales Hospital in Sydney, Australia, consulted on this video along with Dr. Meg Smith, the president of the New South Wales Association for Mental Health and a bipolar herself.

The Devil and Daniel Johnston. DVD, movie/documentary, 2005.

This nonfiction movie/documentary tells the sad yet inspiring story of Daniel Johnston through a treasure-trove of archival footage. We feel for the extremely creative Daniel as his family urges him to set aside his artistic and musical passions to become "useful" and "productive" and "well-rounded." Yet we also sympathize with Daniel's parents, who struggle with this son who disrupts family life and uses their private lives as fodder for his art but always rescue him when he needs help. Daniel's dual diagnosis of bipolar disease and schizophrenia has rendered him chronically mentally ill, yet he maintains a cult following for his art and music.

I Told You I Was Ill: The Life and Legacy of Spike Milligan. Documentary. Done with the cooperation of Milligan's children: spikemilliganlegacy.com.

Spike Milligan has been called the father of British comedy and he influenced Monty Python among other British comics. He cowrote and performed on *The Goon Show* with Peter Sellers and produced numerous books (memoirs, poetry, a comic novel, and children's verse and books) and drawings. Milligan himself appears in the film, talking seriously about his manic-depression and other aspects of his life. His daughter Jane conducts interviews with the people who knew or worked with Milligan, and his brother fills in the gaps of family history. Milligan was bipolar, and, while the details of his mental illness are not heavily featured in this film, you can hear the effects of his depressions on two of his daughters and his coworkers. At one point Milligan recites a poem ("Hope") he wrote about bipolar suicide. Jane seems to be in denial about her father's illness, believing Milligan's hypomanic brilliance was his true nature, but he was in and out of the hospital many times, was psychotic, and once tried to kill Peter Sellers with a potato peeler. Although his family history isn't discussed in this film, research reveals his mother was manic-depressive and he had odd relatives, such as an aunt who put sulphur in her socks to ward off arthritis and left a yellow sulphur trail wherever she went and an uncle who was obsessed by walking as far as he could without opening his eyes.

The Informant! 2009 DVD, starring Matt Damon, based on the book by the same name, by Kurt Eichenwald.

This movie is based on the true story of brilliant and successful senior executive Mark Whitacre, who helped the FBI build a case against his company's worldwide price-fixing operation. Mark, a PhD biochemist who must learn to navigate the business end of the company as he rises in the executive ranks, doesn't approve of price fixing, yet he goes along with what the company requires him to do. He is clearly grandiose and delusional, believing the board of directors will reward his whistle-blowing by making him president of the company. Whitacre's bipolar disease is diagnosed as he worsens under the pressure that ensues for him after the FBI raid his company and he's not seen as the hero he thought he was. Whitacre's bipolar symptoms are downplayed in this movie, but they are there for those that know what to watch for. In particular, his creative thinking, which is just short of racing thoughts, are nicely shown, and his chronic lying exemplifies his delusional frame of mind. Whitacre is now treated for his bipolar disease and is COO of another biotechnology corporation and is currently doing well. He admits that his undiagnosed bipolar disease affected his judgment. He works with a prison ministry and also provides training for FBI agents on how to help untrained undercover agents handle the stress they experience.

My Sister's Keeper. 2002 DVD, *Hallmark Hall of Fame* presentation, based on the book *My Sister's Keeper: Learning to Cope with a Sister's Mental Illness* by Margaret Moorman.

This movie centers on the relationship between two sisters from childhood to adulthood. One leaves home and pursues a successful career in New York City, while the other is chronically mentally ill with bipolar disease, with marked psychosis and struggles to live independently. The mother devotes her life to caring for her mentally ill daughter and sacrifices herself in order for the well daughter to leave home and be "free." The depiction of bipolar disease is accurate albeit a bit simplistic. However, the emotions of the caring but overwhelmed family members and the difficulties in handling a manic, psychotic, or depressed loved one are very realistic. The director of this movie has personal experience with mental illness in his family and it shows.

The Silver Linings Playbook. 2012 DVD of the movie, based on the novel of the same title, written by Matthew Quick.

This movie was based on a novel that was written by a former English teacher with a family history of mental illness, who suffers periodic depressions along with chronic anxiety, and who was suffering from depression when he wrote the book. Although Quick never specifies the mental illness the main character in the book has, the movie screenplay clearly states Pat has bipolar disease; the screenwriter and director has a son with bipolar disease and OCD and he wanted to depict that particular mental illness in the movie. He does so with compassion but also with realism, as others are often afraid or uncomfortable around the mentally ill characters in the movie. This movie shows a family accepting mental illness and learning to adjust and move forward.

Stephen Fry: The Secret Life of the Manic Depressive, Parts 1 and 2. Emmy Award (2000) winning British documentary that can be found at topdocumentaryfilms.com or YouTube.

Stephen Fry was diagnosed with bipolar disease at age 37 after a near-suicide and has suffered extremes of mood all of his life. Fry wanted to learn more about bipolar disease because he recognized his disease was worsening and he needed to make a decision about being medicated. Many bipolar individuals are interviewed, including Carrie Fisher, Richard Dreyfuss and Andy Behrman (Electroboy). A range of bipolar severity is shown and many aspects of the disease are covered. The ending is vague and romanticized and Fry never tells us his final decision about medication. I discovered that he decided against medication because he believed he suffered only from cyclothymia (he calls it "bipolar lite"), despite evidence to the contrary very clearly outlined in this documentary. His decision not to medicate resulted in another suicide attempt in 2012. Fry is no longer in denial about the seriousness of his bipolar disease and is now on medication.

up/down. 2011 documentary, YouTube.

This excellent documentary begins by showing interviews of random people on the street regarding their understanding of bipolar disease. A variety of bipolars are interviewed and discuss their disease in detail, in a question and answer format. All ages are represented and all aspects of the disease are covered. Family members and loved ones are also interviewed. My only criticism is that in the beginning list of famous bipolars, Kurt Vonnegut's name is included. I've found no credible evidence that Vonnegut had bipolar disease, although his son, Mark, has it. Mark clearly states in his current memoir that his disease came from his mother's side of the family.

Bipolar Resource Books

Atkins, Charles. *The Bipolar Disorder Answer Book.* Naperville, IL: Sourcebooks, 2007.

Copeland (PhD), Mary Ellen. *Wellness Recovery Action Plan.* Atlanta: Peach, 2002.

Fawcett (MD), Jan, Bernard Golden (PhD), and Nancy Rosenfeld. *New Hope for People with Bipolar Disorder.* Roseville, California: Prima Health, 2000.

Fink (MD), Candida, and Joe Kraynak. *Bipolar Disorder for Dummies.* Hoboken, NJ: Wiley, 2013.

Miklowitz (PhD), David. *The Bipolar Survivor Guide: What You and Your Family Need to Know.* New York: Guilford, 2011.

Mountain (MD), Jane. *Beyond Bipolar: 7 Steps to Wellness.* Denver: Chapter One, 2008.

_____. *Bipolar Disorder: Insights for Recovery.* Denver: Chapter One, 2008.

Otto (PhD), Michael, et al. *A Guide for Individuals and Families Living with Bipolar Disorder.* New York: Oxford University Press, 2008.

Owen, Sarah, and Amanda Saunders. *Bipolar Disorder: The Ultimate Guide.* Oxford: Oneworld, 2008.

Bipolar Memoirs

Ant, Adam. *Stand and Deliver: The Autobiography.* London: Pan Macmillan, 2006.

This book is a fascinating look at Adam's life and he writes objectively, honestly, and without self-pity about how bipolar disease has both made him who he became and took so much from him at the same time. From his initial suicide attempt in his early twenties to his later breakdowns, diagnosis, repeated failures to comply with his medication schedule and the resultant worsening mood swings, he makes no excuses for his actions and asks for no pity. While a sizable portion of the book chronicles his career, his disease is so intertwined in everything he does during those prolonged years of hypomania that your interest is held throughout the book, even if you've never heard of Adam and the Ants. If Adam's BBC documentary left you wanting to know more about his struggles with bipolar disease, this book will fill in all the gaps.

Behrman, Andy. *Electroboy: A Memoir of Mania*. New York: Random House, 2003.
This book portrays the life of a man who began as a weird, neurotic teen, yet grew into an extremely successful art dealer. It concentrates on the author's life outside his all-consuming day job—his substance abuse, the gay strip clubs he hung out in as well as his involvement in gay male prostitution, his additional businesses on the side, even his airline flights taken on a whim (on an impulse he flew to Germany just to watch the Berlin wall coming down). Even after his diagnosis, he continued to struggle because he lived nearly the same manic lifestyle as he had before, even if his medications had toned him down somewhat. Eventually he gained insight into his bipolar disorder and recognized that his lifestyle had to change in order for him to gain control over his disease. Today, he is married with children and is a suicide prevention and mental health advocate who works to end the stigma of mental illness.

Cheney, Terri. *Manic: A Memoir*. New York: William Morrow, 2008.
If you have ever wanted to get inside the head of a highly functional bipolar to experience mania in all its perturbations, this is the book to read. While Cheney describes depression just as powerfully as she does mania, it's no surprise that all the action revolves around the mania. It's not the action that held my attention, however. It was the thinking and explaining of her manic actions that I found so intriguing as well as the self-control Cheney used to muscle her mania into submission until she got to the point of no control. Only someone with that much willpower would give up a lucrative and high-profile profession for stability, sanity, and a simpler lifestyle of writing and working for mental health causes. Cheney's story is, typically, one of delayed diagnosis (depression), multiple suicide attempts, lack of understanding in her family, and the fear of stigma in both her job and her personal life.

Corrington, Robert S. *Riding the Windhorse: Manic-Depressive Disorder and the Quest for Wholeness*. New York: Hamilton, 2003.
Corrington is an American philosopher and theologian who brings his spiritual and philosophical viewpoint to this book about his bipolar experience. He was raised in a chaotic and unstable home, first with a violent, bipolar mother whose postpartum onset of psychosis after his birth led her to try to kill him, and later with an alcoholic and emotionally and verbally abusive stepmother. His older sister, who protected him from his mother, became chronically mentally ill with bipolar disease and his mother eventually lived on the streets or in a halfway house. Corrington had years of therapy and he feared becoming mentally ill, but he never connected his restlessness or worsening depressions with the disease that afflicted his mother and sister. Because he was diagnosed later in life, he still suffers mood swings despite treatment and works hard to control his bipolar disease. Also included in the book is a case study of Sir Isaac Newton, whom Corrington believes was bipolar.

Duke, Patty, and Gloria Hochman. *A Brilliant Madness: Living with Manic-Depressive Illness*. New York: Bantam, 1987.
You can't help but be touched by the story of Patty Duke, who endured years of emotional upheaval, dragging her family along in her wake and destroying three marriages in the process. It's not that she didn't want help—she did, and she tried every therapy out there—it's that nothing she tried worked. As her disease worsened over time she eventually came to the right diagnosis and began what she calls her wonder drug, lithium, which finally allowed her the stable life she had desperately sought for so many years. Duke's chapters are interspersed with informative chapters written by Hochman, a medical writer who fills in the medical facts about bipolar disease. While some of the medical information is out of date (the book was updated in 1992), this book presents an inspiring story of successful treatment with a decidedly happy ending.

Fisher, Carrie. *Wishful Drinking.* New York: Simon & Schuster, 2008.

This is a short, easy read about growing up among celebrities in Hollywood. Fisher explains how bipolar behavior is not only overlooked but celebrated in Hollywood, as long as it stays under some measure of control or kept hidden from the public. Fisher's words and clever, self deprecating humor display a bipolar's talent for writing and word usage. Her account of her hospitalization for acute mania, while brief, is funny yet desperate. She frankly discusses electroconvulsive therapy (ECT), which has destroyed her memory but successfully treats her bipolar disease. She claims to have written this book so she will have a written record of what her one-woman show is all about, in case she forgets. While you may finish this book wishing for more details about Fisher's bipolar disease, you are left with a good understanding of how her bipolar disease has shaped her talent, her personality, and her life. Fisher does make a mistake in her book, confusing bipolar-I with bipolar-II, claiming she has the worse form of bipolar disease, which she calls bipolar-II rather than bipolar-I. With two psychiatric hospitalizations for psychotic mania under her belt, Fisher is most definitely bipolar-I.

Greenberg, Michael. *Hurry Down Sunshine: A Father's Story of Love and Madness.* New York: Vintage, 2008.

This book chronicles the acute manic and psychotic attack of the author's 15-year-old daughter, Sally, during the summer of 1996. Written from a disbelieving and scared father's point of view, the experiences and emotions of the loving extended family are raw and real. Because no one educates this family about Sally's bipolar disease, everyone but the stepmother looks for something or someone to blame. There are tantalizing hints throughout the book about this or that family member who might be on the bipolar spectrum but Greenberg never gives enough details for the reader to know for sure. He keeps the focus on the day-to-day details of dealing with an acutely mentally ill person in the household; the financial, mental and emotional strain is tremendous. A postscript to the book lets the reader know what Sally is doing today.

Hornbacher, Marya. *Madness.* Boston: Mariner, reprint. ed., 2009.

Born to a family with a long history of mental illness, Hornbacher's severe and persistent symptoms began early. She was self-medicating with alcohol at age 10, promiscuous by age 14, bulimic by her late teens, and cutting herself by her twenties. She was finally diagnosed with rapidly cycling bipolar disease at age 24 and responded to medication, although she continued to deny her diagnosis for quite some time. This book does a particularly good job of describing the details of bipolar attacks as well as what it's like to be a bipolar child. There are years of frequent mental hospitalizations (every few months) that eventually become less frequent as Hornbacher gets better at managing her illness. She is a very brittle bipolar, but in the end she manages her disease with tight-fisted control.

Jamison, Kay Redfield. *An Unquiet Mind.* New York: First Vintage, 2006.

Jamison is a clinical professor of psychiatry at Johns Hopkins University School of Medicine and an expert on mood disorders, so this account of her personal struggle with bipolar disease is particularly compelling. When we learn that she stopped her medication multiple times, even though she understands more about the disease than most of us ever will, it shows us that bipolars make the same mistakes, no matter who they are. Jamison is able to brilliantly describe what it's like to be bipolar and how it affected her personal and professional life and drove her to the brink of suicide. This book is a must-read for all bipolars.

Kazmierczak, Jeff D. *Neural Misfire: A True Story of Manic Depression.* Chicago: Koda Services, 2000.

This book is a fictionalized account of the author's bipolar disorder, beginning dramatically with the 18-year-old main character's incarceration for reckless driving during full-blown mania and then backtracking nine months to demonstrate the build-up of symptoms that led to that crisis. Private thoughts are set apart by the use of italics so the reader can better understand the bipolar thinking that lies behind the main character's actions or spoken words. His world begins to fall apart as he becomes aggressive and then violent, is hospitalized, escapes, is sent home, threatens his parents in order to extort money from them, and is eventually arrested for the reckless driving that opens the book. A court mandated hospitalization results in the bipolar diagnosis. The epilogue, set one year later, rang a false note with me. Most bipolars have barely recovered from a bad attack at that point, much less have the perspective the young man claims to have gained on life as a result of his breakdown. This is a minor flaw, however. The book is worth reading simply for the insight it affords into the slow progression of bipolar symptoms and how difficult it can be for parents, friends, and school authorities to recognize when eccentric behavior crosses the line into mental illness.

McCarter, Melissa Miles. *Insanity: A Love Story*. Ironton, MO: CreateSpace, 2009.

McCarter is a writer and a graduate student working on her doctorate in rhetoric and composition. Her book deals with the story of her mental illness, which required hospitalization during a psychotic episode that ultimately resulted in the diagnosis of bipolar disorder. While this book contains scattered typographical or grammatical errors, if you can overlook those flaws, the insight it affords into the surprisingly sane mind of one deemed insane is invaluable. McCarter's struggle with her delusions and how she ultimately learns to live with them reflects the current psychiatric struggle over where to draw the line regarding sanity: should all delusions be gone or can they still be present but not acted upon?

Styron, William. *Darkness Visible: A Memoir of Madness*. New York: Vintage, 1990.

This book began as a lecture on affective (mood) disorders and was expanded to book form. Beautifully written by this Pulitzer Prize winning author of *The Confessions of Nat Turner* and *Sophie's Choice*, this short book is considered one of the classic texts on depression. Styron's depression began at 60 when he stopped drinking. While he claims to have never been depressed in the past, he later recognizes that his literature was filled with depression, doom and suicide, that his father had suffered from chronic depression and had been hospitalized for a breakdown when Styron was a child, and that Styron himself had suffered irritable and discontented times in his life when he was unable to write, which magnified his alcohol use. Antidepressant therapy during his hospitalization made him "edgy" and "disagreeably hyperactive" (54) and he never found an antidepressant that worked. He suffered a second, severe psychotic depression 15 years later after what his wife described as periods of ups and downs, with speeches and writing done during that time that she believed were the best of his career. This is enough evidence to include Styron in the bipolar category.

Sutherland, Stuart. *Breakdown: A Personal Crisis and a Medical Dilemma*. Pinter & Martin, 2010.

Sutherland is a psychologist who was plunged into a severe depression when he discovered that his wife was having an affair with his long-time friend. He was eventually hospitalized and treated. After a few months he flipped into three months of hypomania. Thereafter he suffered the mood swings of a bipolar, becoming depressed in the summer and hypomanic in the winter, but none of his subsequent mood swings were as pronounced as his original depression and hypomania, thanks to proper treatment. He is adamant that, except for his first depression, none of his mood swings were caused by any external event. He and his wife eventually separated due to her continued affairs; although when he was hypomanic, Sutherland was hypersexual, seducing women in front of his wife and pretending, he claims, to seduce both homosexual and heterosexual men. The original version of this book was written in 1976, with updates in following years, and is brutally frank during a time when no one openly talked about mental illness. It paved the way for the bipolar memoirs of the future.

Wolpert, Lewis. *Malignant Sadness*. London: Faber & Faber: 2006.

Wolpert is a developmental biologist who was hospitalized for a severe suicidal depression that he said was worse than watching his wife die from cancer. After he wrote the book, he had four more episodes, although none were as severe as his initial one, thanks to quicker treatment. His depressions were marked by severe anxiety, panic attacks, and multiple physical symptoms. Cognitive behavior therapy was helpful, but a brief attempt at psychoanalysis, at his wife's insistence, was useless. Antidepressants worked for Wolpert but made him anxious and irritable and when he recovered he said he was "mildly more manic ... a little more reckless" than normal (162). His agitated depressions and his hypomania when the depressions lifted point to a diagnosis of bipolar-II, which was unknown at that time. He explores depression from all viewpoints in this book. Some of the information is outdated, as it was originally written in 1999, but the book is worth reading for the description of depression from the male point of view.

Works Cited

"ACT Model." *ACT Association.* Assertive Community Treatment Association. 21 Mar. 2007. Web. 25 Aug. 2013.

"Actress Jenifer Lewis Puts a New Face on Bipolar Disease." BET.com. Black Entertainment Television. 20 Jun. 2008. Web. 22 Aug. 2013.

Adam Ant: The Madness of Prince Charming. BBC Documentary. 2004. Web. 28 Aug. 2013.

"Agent: Robbins Has Bipolar Disorder." SI.com. Associated Press. 03 Feb. 2003. Web. 22 Aug. 2013.

Akiskal, H.S. "The Emergence of the Bipolar Spectrum: Validation Along Clinical-Epidemiologic and Familial-Genetic Lines." *Psychopharmacol Bull* 40.4 (2008): 99–115. Web. 18 Aug. 2013.

Akiskal, H.S., M. Bourgeois, and J. Angst, et al. "Re-evaluating the Prevalence of and Diagnostic Composition Within the Broad Clinical Spectrum of Bipolar Disorders." *J Affect Disord* 59 Suppl 1(2000): s5–s30. Web. 18 Aug. 2013.

Akiskal, H.S., R.H. Rosenthal, and T.L. Rosenthal, et al. "Differentiation of Primary Affective Illness from Situational, Symptomatic, and Secondary Depressions." *Arch Gen Psychiatry* 36.6 (1979): 635–43. Web. 18 Aug. 2013.

American Psychiatric Association. *Desk Reference to the Diagnostic Criteria from "DSM-V."* Washington, DC: American Psychiatric, 2013. Print.

Amminger, G.P., M.R. Schäfer, and K. Papageorgiou, et al. "Long-Chain Omega–3 Fatty Acids for Indicated Prevention of Psychotic Disorders: A Randomized, Placebo-Controlled Trial." *Arch Gen Psychiatry* 67.2 (2010): 146–54. Web. 25 Aug. 2013.

Andreasen, Nancy C. *The Creating Brain: The Neuroscience of Genius.* New York: Dana, 2005. Print.

_____. "Creativity and Mental Illness: Prevalence Rates in Writers and Their First Degree Relatives." *Am J Psychiatry* 144.10 (1987): 1288–92. Web. 18 Aug. 2013.

Ant, Adam. *Stand and Deliver: The Autobiography.* London: Pan Macmillan, 2006. Print.

Apter, Jeff. *Fornication: The Red Hot Chili Peppers Story.* London: Omnibus, 2005. Print.

Baldessarini, R.J., and J. Hennen. "Genetics of Suicide: An Overview." *Harv Rev Psychiatry* 12.1 (2004): 1–13. Web. 15 Aug. 2013.

Baldoni, John. "Mike Wallace: Fighting the Good Fight." *CBS MoneyWatch.* CBS News. 10 April 2012. Web. 22 Aug. 2013.

Barnett, J.H., and J.W. Smoller. "The Genetics of Bipolar Disorder." *Neuroscience* 164.1 (2009): 331–43. Web. 17 Aug. 2013.

Bauer, M.S., G.E. Simon, and E. Ludman, et al. "Bipolarity in Bipolar Disorder: Distribution of Manic and Depressive Symptoms in a Treated Population." *Br J Psychiatry* 187 (2005): 87–88. Web. 27 Aug. 2013.

Baum, A.E., N. Akula, and M. Cabanero, et al. "A Genome-Wide Association Study Implicates

Diacylglycerol Kinase Eta (DGKH) and Several Other Genes in the Etiology of Bipolar Disorder." *Mol Psychiatry* 13.2 (2–8): 197–207. Web. 17 Aug. 2013.

Behrman, Andy. *Electroboy: A Memoir of Mania.* New York: Random, 2003. Print.

Bell, Quentin. *Virginia Woolf: A Biography.* New York: Harcourt Brace Jovanovich, 1972. Print.

Benson, Heidi. "Historian Iris Chang Won Many Battles; The War She Lost Raged Within." *SFGate.* Hearst Communications. 17 Apr. 2005. Web. 22 Aug. 2013.

Berger, Ken. "West Deals with Bipolar Disorder, Gets Back on Track." *CBSSports.* CBS Broadcasting. 22 Nov. 2010. Web. 22 Aug. 2013.

Bertelsen, A., B. Harvald, and M. Hauge. "A Danish Twin Study of Manic-Depressive Disorders." *Br J Psychiatry* 130 (1977): 330–51. Web. 17 Aug. 2013.

Blehar, M.C., J.R. DePaulo, Jr., and E.S. Gershon, et al. "Women with Bipolar Disorder: Findings from the NIMH Genetics Initiative Sample." *Psychopharmacology Bulletin* 34.3 (1998): 239–43. Web. 15 Aug. 2013.

Borden, Timothy. "Darryl Strawberry." *encyclopedia.com.* High Beam Research. 2004. Web. 22 Aug. 2013.

Brand, Russell. *My Booky Wook: A Memoir of Sex, Drugs, and Stand-Up.* New York: Collins, 2009. Print.

Brauser, Deborah. "APA Answers DSM-5 Critics." *Medscape.* WebMD LLC. 9 Nov. 2011. Web. 28 Aug. 2013.

Bray, Elisa. "Interview: Sinead O'Connor." *eMusic.* ROVI. 21 Feb. 2012. Web. 2 Aug. 2013.

Brockes, Emma. "The Emma Brockes Interview: Frank Bruno." *theguardian.* Guardian News and Media. 23 Oct. 2005. Web. 22 Aug. 2013.

Brown, David. *Tchaikovsky: The Man and His Music.* New York: First Pegasus, 2009. Print.

Caramagno, Thomas C. *The Flight of Mind: Virginia Woolf's Art and Manic-Depressive Illness.* Berkeley: University of California Press, 1992. Print.

Caruso, Kevin. "*Harry Potter* Author J.K. Rowling: 'I Considered Suicide.'" Suicide.org. n.p. n.d. Web. 28 Aug. 2013.

Cheney, Terri. *Manic: A Memoir.* New York: William Morrow, 2008. Print.

Chiaroni, P., E.S. Hantouche, and J. Gouvernet, et al. "The Cyclothymic Temperament in Healthy Controls and Familially At Risk Individuals for Mood Disorder: Endophenotype for Genetic Studies?" *J Affect Dis* 85.1–2 (2005):135–45 Web. 18 Aug. 2013.

Cichon, S., T.W. Muhleisen, and F.A. Degenhardt, et al. "Genome-Wide Association Study Identifies Genetic Variation in Neurocan as a Susceptibility Factor for Bipolar Disorder." *Am J Hum Genet* 88.3 (2011): 372–81. Web. 17 Aug. 2013.

Clerk, Carol. *Saga of Hawkwind.* London: Omnibus, 2004.

Clooney, Rosemary, and Raymond Strait. *This for Remembrance: The Autobiography of Rosemary Clooney, an Irish-American Singer.* Chicago: Playboy, 1977. Prints.

Cohen, L.S. "Treatment of Bipolar Disorder During Pregnancy." *J Clin Psychiatry* 68. Suppl. 9 (2007): 4–9. Web. 16 Aug. 2013.

Collins, Nick. "Raoul Moat: Gazza Arrives in Rothbury to 'Offer His Support.'" London *Daily Telegraph.* Telegraph Media Group. 09 Jul. 2010. Web. 22 Aug. 2013.

Columbus, Christopher. *The Libro de las profecias of Christopher Columbus.* Translated by Delno C. West and August Kling. Gainesville: University of Florida Press, 1992. Print.

_____. *The Log of Christopher Columbus.* Translated by Robert Fulson. Camden, ME: International, 1987. Print.

_____. *The Voyage of Christopher Columbus: Columbus' Own Journal of Discovery.* Translated by John Cummins. New York: St. Martin's, 1992. Print.

Copeland, M.E. *Wellness Recovery Action Plan,* Atlanta: Peach, 2002. Print.

Corrington, Robert S. *Riding the Windhorse: Manic-Depressive Disorder and the Quest for Wholeness.* New York: Hamilton, 2003. Print.

Demarr, Mary J. *Kaye Gibbons: A Critical Companion.* Westport, CT: Greenwood, 2003. Print.

Dias, R.S., B. Lafer, and C. Russo, et al. "Longitudinal Follow-up of Bipolar Disorder in

Women with Premenstrual Exacerbation: Findings from STEP-BD." *Am J Psychiatry* 168.4 (2011): 386–94. Web. 15 Aug. 2013.

Dickinson, Emily. *The Letters of Emily Dickinson.* Vols. 1–3. Edited by T.H. Johnson and T. Ward. Cambridge, MA: Harvard University, 1958.

"Did Florence Nightingale Suffer from Bipolar Disorder?" *Medical News Today.* MediLexicon, Intl. 18 Apr. 2004. Web. 22 Aug. 2013.

Dos Santos, Kristin. "Hugh Laurie Speaks Candidly About His Struggle with Depression." *Celebrities with Diseases.* 05 Jan. 2010. Wikimedia. Web. 22 Aug. 2013.

Dowell, Pat. "Jonathan Winters Reflects on a Lifetime of Laughs." NPR. Disqus. 30 Jul. 2011. Web. 22 Aug. 2011.

Duke, Patty. *Brilliant Madness: Living with Manic Depression.* New York: Bantam, 1987. Print.

Eby, Douglas. "Amy Tan and Writing and Depression." *The Creative Mind.* PsychCentral. 19 Sep. 2010. Web. 21 Aug. 2013.

Erikson, Erik. *Young Man Luther: A Study in Psychoanalysis and History.* New York: Norton, 1993. Print.

Ferreira, M.A., M.C. O'Donovan, and Y.A. Meng, et al. "Collaborative Genome-Wide Association Analysis Supports a Role for ANK3 and CACNA1C in Bipolar Disorder." *Nat Genet* 40.9 (2008):1056–58. Web. 17 Aug. 2013.

Fisher, Carrie. *Wishful Drinking.* New York: Simon & Schuster, 2008. Print.

Frank, Ellen. *Treating Bipolar Disorder: A Clinician's Guide to Interpersonal and Social Rhythm Therapy.* New York: Guilford, 2005. Print.

Gallagher, James. "Stephen Fry: Suicide Risk in Bipolar Disorder." *BBC News Health.* BBC. 6 June 2013. Web. 22 Aug. 2013.

Gartner, John. *The Hypomanic Edge: The Link Between (a Little) Craziness and (a Lot of) Success in America.* New York: Simon & Schuster, 2005. Print.

Gascoigne, Paul. *Being Gazza: Tackling My Demons.* London: Headline, 2006. Print.

_____. *Gazza: My Story.* London: Headline, 2004. Print.

Gershon, E.S., J. Hamovit, and J.J. Guroff, et al. "A Family Study of Schizoaffective, Bipolar I, Bipolar II, Unipolar, and Normal Probands." *Arch Gen Psychiatry* 39.10 (1982): 1157–67. Web. 17 Aug. 2013.

Ghaemi, Nassir. *A First Rate Madness: Uncovering the Links Between Leadership and Mental Illness.* London: Penguin, 2011. Print.

Gitlin, M.J., J. Swendsen, and T.L. Heller, et al. "Relapse and Impairment in Bipolar." *Am J Psychiatry* 152.11 (1995):1635–40. Web. 24 Aug. 2013.

Goldberg, J.P. *Bipolar Disorders: Clinical Course and Outcome.* Washington, DC: American Psychiatric Press, 1999. Print.

Goodwin, Frederick K., and Kay R. Jamison. *Manic-Depressive Illness: Bipolar Disorders and Recurrent Depression.* 2 vols. New York: Oxford University Press, 2007. Print.

Goodwin, Gloria. "Winona Ryder's Battle with Anxiety and Depression." *Beyond Anxiety and Depression.* n.p. 23 Jan. 2012. Web. 22 Aug. 2013.

Graham, Katherine. *Personal History.* New York: Knopf, 1997.

Greenburg, Michael. *Hurry Down Sunshine: A Father's Story of Love and Madness.* New York: Vintage, 2008.

Hardy, Rebecca. "A Kinks Reunion? Never!" Dailymail. Associated Newspapers. 31 Oct. 2010. Web. 21 Aug. 2013.

Harmon, Melissa B. "Tchaikovsky: The Tormented Life of a Musical Genius." *Biography.* Dec. 2002: 94–95,106,108. Print.

Hershman, Jablow D., and Julian Lieb. *Manic Depression and Creativity.* New York: Prometheus, 1998. Print.

Holden, Anthony. *Laurence Olivier.* New York: Atheneum, 1988. Print.

Horan, Michael. "Hay Reveals Pain of Bipolar." *Herald Sun.* News Ltd. 29 Aug. 2006. Web. 22 Aug. 2013.

Hornbacher, Marya. *Madness: A Bipolar Life.* New York: First Mariner, 2008. Print.

"Hungarian Research Postulates Syd Barrett Had Genetic Condition." Sydbarrettpinkfloyd. com. n.p. 21 Jul. 2009. Web. 28 Aug. 2013.

International Schizophrenia Consortium, S.M. Purcell, N.R. Wray, et al. "Common Polygenic Variation Contributes to Risk of Schizophrenia and Bipolar Disorder." *Nature* 460.7256 (2009): 748–52. Web. 17 Aug. 2013.

"Interview with Author Marya Hornbacher." Ask a Bipolar. *askabipolarwww.* 5 Jun. 2011. Web. 30 Aug. 2013.

James, Del. "The World According to W. Axl Rose." Heretodaygonetohell.com. HTGTH. April 1989. Web. 28 Aug. 2013.

James, Sallie. "Underwood Runs into Traffic." SunSentinel. 06 Jan. 2001. Web. 28 Aug. 2013.

James, William. *The Varieties of Religious Experience: A Study in Human Nature.* New York: Mentor, 1958. Print.

Jamison, Kay R. *Exuberance: The Passion for Life.* New York: Knopf, 2005. Print.

_____. "Mood Disorders and Seasonal Patterns in British Writers and Artists." *Psychiatry* 52.2 (1989): 125–34. Web. 18 Aug. 2013.

_____. *Night Falls Fast: Understanding Suicide.* New York: Vintage, 1999. Print.

_____. *Touched with Fire: Manic-Depressive Illness and the Artistic Temperament.* New York: Simon & Schuster, 1994. Print.

_____. *An Unquiet Mind: A Memoir of Moods and Madness.* New York: First Vintage, 2006. Print.

Jenkins, Joe. "Mike Tyson and Evander Holyfield Trade Jokes About Infamous Ear-Biting Incident on Twitter." *NYDailyNews.* 29 Jun. 2012. Web. 22 Aug. 2013.

Jette, N., S. Patten, and J. Williams, et al. "Comorbidity of Migraine and Psychiatric Disorders—A National Population-Based Study." *Headache* 48.4 (2008): 501–16. Web. 16 Aug. 2013.

Jezer, Marty. *Abbie Hoffman: American Rebel.* New Jersey: Rutgers University Press: 1993. Print.

Kahl, K.G., L. Winter, and U. Schweiger. "The Third Wave of Cognitive Behavioural Therapies." *Curr Opin Psychiatry* 25.6 (2012): 522–28. Web. 25 Aug. 2013.

Karlsson, L.L. "Genetic Association of Giftedness and Creativity with Schizophrenia." *Hereditas* 66.2 (1970): 177–82) Web. 18. Aug. 2013.

Keri, Szaboles. "Genes for Psychosis and Creativity: A Promoter Polymorphism of the Neuregulin 1 Gene Is Related to Creativity in People with High Intellectual Achievement." *Psychol Sci* 20.9 (2009): 1070–73. Web. 24 Aug. 2013.

Khazaee, Malek K. "The Case of Nietzsche's Madness." Existenz 3, no. 1 (Spring 2008). Philosophy Gateway. Web. 28 Aug. 2013.

Kliff, Sarah. "Owen Wilson: Depression." *The Daily Beast.* Newsweek. 13 Oct. 2007. Web. 22 Aug. 2013.

Kraepelin, Emil. *Manic-Depressive Insanity and Paranoia.* Edinburgh: E & S Livingstone, 1921. *Open Library.* Web. 15 August 2013.

"Kristy McNichol." NNDB. Soylent Communications. n.p. Web. 22 Aug. 2013.

Kurtz, Jason. "Ted Turner: I Lost Jane ... I Lost My Job Here ... I Lost My Fortune, Most of It." CNN. 3 May 2012 Web. 19 Aug. 2013.

Kyaga, Simon, Paul Liechtenstein, and Marcus Boman, et al. "Creativity and Mental Disorder: Family Study of 300,000 People with Severe Mental Disorder." *Br. J Psychiatry* 199.5 (2011): 373–39. Web. 24 Aug. 2013.

Landau, Elizabeth. "Hemingway Family Mental Illness Explored in New Film." CNN. 23 Jan. 2013. Web. 22 Aug. 2013.

"Larry King Live Panel Discusses Depression: Transcript." CNN. 12 Jun. 2005. Web. 28 Aug. 2013.

Leonard, Elizabeth. "Carrie Fisher Describes Her Bipolar Crisis." *People.* Time. 14 Mar. 2013. Web. 22 Aug. 2013.

Leung, Rebecca. "Carrey: "Life Is Too Beautiful.'" *60 Minutes*. CBS News. 11 Feb. 2009. Web. 22 Aug. 2013.

Libby, Brian. "Even in His Youth." *HealthDay*. LimeHealth. 11 March 2013. Web. 21 Aug. 2013.

"Linda Hamilton Says She Has Bipolar Disorder." *Today*. NBC News. 14 Sept. 2004. Web. 22 Aug. 2013.

Locke, Colleen. "Body of Missing Boulder Man Found in Hawaii." 9Newswww. Gannett. 14 Jul. 2008. Web. 22 Aug. 2013.

Luoma, J.B., C.E. Martin, and J.L. Pearson. "Contact with Mental Health and Primary Care Providers Before Suicide: A Review of the Evidence." *Am. J. Psychiatry* 159.6 (2002): 909–16. Web. 15 Aug. 2013.

MacCabe, J.H., M.P. Lambe, and P.C. Sham, et al., "Excellent School Performance at age 16 and Risk of Adult Bipolar Disorder: National Cohort Study." *Br J of Psychiatry* 196.2 (2010): 109–15. Web. 18 Aug. 2013.

The Madness of Prince Charming. Adam Ant. BBC Documentary, 2004. Web.

"Margaret Trudeau Reveals Struggle with Bipolar Disorder." *CBCNews*. CBC Radio Canada. 6 May 2006. Web. 22 Aug. 2013.

Matthews, Charles. "The Atom Bomb's Tragic Hero." *HistoryAccess. San Jose Mercury News*. 2005. Web. 22 Aug. 2013.

McCarter, Melissa. *Insanity: A Love Story; A Memoir of Madness and Mania*. CreateSpace, 2009. eBook.

McClymont, Kate, Ellen Connolly, and Malcolm Brown. "Rivkin Children Silent About Fabulously Flawed Father." *Sydney Morning Herald*. Fairfax Media. 3 May 2005. Web. 22 Aug. 2013.

McDermott, John F. "Emily Dickinson Revisited: A Study of Periodicity in Her Work." *Am J Psychiatry* 158.5 (2001): 686–90. Web. 21 Aug. 2013.

McNeil, T.F. "Prebirth and Postbirth Influence on the Relationship Between Creative Ability and Recorded Mental Illness." *J Pers* 39.3 (1971): 391–406. Web. 18 Aug. 2013.

Mendlewicz, J., and J.D. Rainer. "Adoption Study Supporting Genetic Transmission in Manic-Depressive Illness." *Nature* 268.5618 (1977): 327–29. Web. 17 Aug. 2013.

Miklowitz, David. *The Bipolar Disorder Survivor Guide: What You and Your Family Need to Know*. New York: Guilford, 2011. Print.

Moon, Troy. "Meet the Real Informant!" *Pensacola News Journal*. Gannett. 23 Sept. 2009. Web. 22 Aug. 2013.

Morris, Kerry. New York State Writers Institute Seminar Transcript with Kaye Gibbons on 23 Apr. 1998. *Writers Online* 5, no. 1 (Fall 2000). Web. 20 Aug. 2013.

Mountain, Jane. *Bipolar Disorder: Insights for Recovery*. Denver: Chapter One, 2008. Print.

Mueser, Kim T., P.W. Corrigan, and D.W. Hilton, et al. "Illness Management and Recovery: A Review of the Research." *Psychiatr Serv* 53.10 (2002): 1272–84. Web. 25 Aug. 2013.

Murray, Elicia, Maddox, Garry. "Mel Gibson Talks About Being Diagnosed as Bipolar in a New Documentary About the NIDA Acting Class of 1977." *Sydney Morning Herald*. Fairfax Digital. 15 May 2008. Web. 22 Aug. 2013.

O'Connor, J.J., and E.F. Robertson. "Ludwig Boltzmann." history.mcs.st-andrews. School of Mathematic and Statistics, University of St. Andrews, Scotland. Sept. 1998. Web. 22 Aug. 2013.

Oliver, Myrna. "Dr. Hyman Engleberg, 92; Marilyn Monroe's Personal Physician." *Los Angeles Times*. 21 Dec. 2005. Web. 22 Aug. 2013.

Pagett, Nicola, and Graham Swannell. *Diamonds Behind My Eyes*. London: Victor Gollancz, 1998. Print.

Painton, Priscilla. "The Taming of Ted Turner." *Time*. 06 Jan. 1992. Web. 19 Aug. 2013.

Panter, Barry. *Creativity and Madness*. Burbank: Aimed, 1995. Print.

"Paul Gascoigne in Intensive Care in Arizona Hospital After Reacting Badly to Detox Treatment for Alcoholism." London *Daily Telegraph*. Telegraph Media Group. 10 Feb. 2013. Web. 22 Aug. 2013.

"Paul Gascoigne: What Gazza Did Next." *Independent.* Independent Co. 18 Sept. 2006. Web. 22 Aug. 2013.

Pauley, Jane. *Skywriting: A Life Out of the Blue.* New York: Ballantine, 2005. Print.

Peat, David F. *Infinite Potential: The Life and Times of David Bohm.* Reading, MA: Addison Wesley, 1997. Print.

Perugi, G., H.S. Akiskal, and C. Micheli, et al. "The Soft Bipolar Spectrum Redefined: Focus on the Anxious-Sensitive, Impulse-Dyscontrol and Binge-Eating Connection in Bipolar II and Related Conditions." *Psychiatr Clin North Am* 25.4 (2002): 713–37. Web. 18 Aug. 2013.

Petridis, Alexis. "The Astonishing Genius of Brian Wilson." *theguardian.* Guardian News. 24 Jun. 2011. Web. 21 Aug. 2013.

Plato. *Phaedrus and Letters.* Vols. 7, 8. Translated by Walter Hamilton. Great Britain: Hazell, Watson, & Viney, 1973. Print.

Purse, Marcia. "Jean-Claude Van Damme." About.com Bipolar. n.p. 23 Aug. 2012. Web. 22 Aug. 2013.

_____. "Ned Beatty." About.com Bipolar. n.p. 13 Apr. 2005. Web. 22 Aug. 2013.

Richards, R.L., D.K. Kinney, and I. Lunde, et al. "Creativity in Manic-Depression, Cyclothymes, Their Normal Relatives, and Control Subjects." *J Abnorm Psychol* 97.3 (1988): 281–88. Web. 18 Aug. 2013.

Roe, Nicholas. "Against All Odds." London *Daily Telegraph.* Telegraph Media Group. 09 Jun. 2007. Web. 22 Aug. 2013.

Rose, Phyllis. *Woman of Letters: A Life of Virginia Woolf.* New York: Harcourt Brace Jovanovich, 1987. Print.

Rufus, Anneli. "Bipolar Disorder Plays Role in Patricia Cornwell's Financial Melee." *Stuck.* Psychology Today. 22 Oct. 2009. Web. 21 Aug. 2013.

Salahi, Lara. "Amy Winehouse: Career Shadowed by Manic Depression." *ABC News.* World News. 25 Jul. 2011. Web. 21 Aug. 2013.

_____. "Catherine Zeta-Jones Sheds Light on Bipolar II Disorder." *ABC News.* Yahoo News. 14 April 2011. Web. 22 Aug. 2013.

Sarris, J., D. Mischoulon, and I. Schweitzer. "Omega-3 for Bipolar Disorder: Meta-Analyses of Use in Mania and Bipolar Depression." *J Clin Psychiatry* 73.1 (2012): 81–86. Web. 25 Aug. 2013.

Schimelpfening, Nancy. "Pete Wentz Admits He Has Bipolar Disorder." About.com. Depression. n.p. Web. 21 Aug. 2013.

Schottle, Daniel, C.G Huber, and T. Bock, et al. "Psychotherapy for Bipolar: A Review of the Most Recent Studies." *Curr Opin Psychiatry* 24.6 (2011): 549–555. Web. 25 Aug. 2013.

Sellers, Patricia. "Ted Turner Is a Worried Man." *Fortune.* CNN Money. 26 May 2003. Web. 19 Aug. 2013.

Shih, R.A., P.L. Belmonte, and P.P. Zandi. "A Review of the Evidence from Family, Twin and Adoption Studies for a Genetic Contribution to Adult Psychiatric Disorders." *Int Rev Psychiatry* 16.4 (2004):260–83. Web. 18 Aug. 2013.

Shorter, E., and D. Healy. *A History of Electroconvulsive Treatment in Mental Illness.* New Brunswick, NJ: Rutgers University Press, 2007. Print.

"Slater Reveals Bipolar Illness." theage.com. Age Company. 14 Mar. 2005. Web. 22 Aug. 2013.

Smith, Barbara Peters. "Richard Dreyfuss Talks About Living with Bipolar Disorder." *Herald Tribune Health.* Herald-Tribune. 3 Apr. 2012. Web. 22 Aug. 2013.

Starkey, Ed. *My Life—My Way: "Frank 'Ol' Blue Eyes' Sinatra."* Bloomington, IN: Author House, 2008. Print.

Steadman, Keith A. *The Bipolar Expeditionist.* Bloomington, IL: iUniverse, 2008. Print.

Stephen Fry: The Secret Life of the Manic Depressive. Perf. Stephen Fry. 2006. BBC Documentary. Web. 25 Aug. 2013.

Stewart, Rob. "The Life and Times of Paul Gascoigne." London *Daily Telegraph.* Telegraph Media Group. 14 Feb. 2008. Web. 22 Aug. 2013.

Stossel, John, and Andrew Sullivan. "Winners: Drew Carey's Inspiring Journey." *ABC News.* Yahoo News. 14 Nov. 2007. Web. 22 Aug. 2013.

Styron, William. *Darkness Visible: A Memoir of Madness.* New York: Vintage, 1990. Print.

Sutherland, Stuart. *Breakdown: A Personal Crisis and a Medical Dilemma.* London: Pinter & Martin, 2010. Print.

Szalavitz, Maia. "Jesse Jackson Jr.'s Bipolar 2: A Diagnosis Muddle by the Market." *Time Health and Family.* Time Web. 16 Aug. 2012. 27 Aug. 2013.

Tank, Ron. "Burgess Meredith Dies at 89." CNN. Cable News Network.10 Sep. 1997. Web. 28 Aug. 2013.

Taviani, Paolo Emilio. *Columbus: The Great Adventure; His Life, His Times, and His Voyages.* New York: Orion, 1991. Print.

Tchaikovsky, Modest. *The Life and Letters of Peter Ilich Tchaikovsky.* New York: John Lane, 1906. Ebook.

"Tim Smith Leaving Eels to Battle Bipolar." kickoff.net. Australian Associated Press. 14 Apr. 2008. Web. 22 Aug. 2013.

Toole, Betty A. *Ada: The Enchantress of Numbers; Poetical Science.* Metuchen, NJ: Strawberry, 1998. Print.

Turner, Ted, and Bill Burke. *Call Me Ted.* New York: Hatchette, 2008. Print.

Urquhart, Alasdair. "Emil Post." *Handbook of the History of Logic: Logic from Russell to Church.* Vol. 5. Edited by Dov. M. Gabbay and John Woods. Amsterdam: North Holland, 2009. 617- 66. Print.

Viguera, A.C., T. Whitfield, and R.J. Baldessarini, et al. "Risk of Recurrence in Women with Bipolar Disorder During Pregnancy: Prospective Study of Mood Stabilizer Discontinuation." *Am J Psychiatry* 164.12 (2007): 1817–24. Web. 16 Aug. 2013.

Vonnegut, Mark. *Just Like Someone Without Mental Illness Only More So.* New York: Bantam, 2011. Print.

Wachtler, Sol. *After the Madness: A Judge's Memoir of His Time in Prison.* New York: Random House, 1997. Print.

Waggoner, Martha. "Novelist Kaye Gibbons Faces Yet Another Hurdle." *Reading Eagle.* Associated Press. 20 June 2009. Web. 20 Aug. 2013.

Walker, Marion "Author Kaye Gibbons Pleads Guilty in Drug Case." *USA Today.* Gannett. 10 Mar. 2009. Web. 20 Aug. 2013.

Weaver, Clair. "Joey Johns' Bipolar Despair." London *Daily Telegraph.* Telegraph Media Group. 02 Sept. 2007. Web. 22 Aug. 2013.

"Wellness Recovery Action Plan (WRAP)." NREPP SAMHSA.gov. USA.gov. 15 May 2013. Web. 25 Aug. 2013.

Willcutt, E., and M. McQueen. "Genetic and Environmental Vulnerability to Bipolar Spectrum Disorder." In *Understanding Bipolar Disorder: A Developmental Psychological Perspective.* Edited by J.D. Miklowitz and D. Cicchetti. New York: Guilford, 2010. Print.

Williams, Alex. "Vanishing Act." *New York Magazine.* New York Media. 02 Feb. 2004. Web. 22 Aug. 2013.

Wolpert, Lewis. *Malignant Sadness.* London: Faber, 2006. Print.

Woolf, Leonard. *Beginning Again: An Autobiography of the Years 1911–1918.* New York: Harcourt Brace Jovanovich, 1964. Print.

Woolf, Virginia. *The Diary of Virginia Woolf.* 5 vols. Edited by Anne Olivier Bell and Andrew McNeilie. New York: Harcourt Brace Jovanovich, 1976–84. Print.

_____. *The Letters of Virginia Woolf.* 6 vols. Edited by Nigel Nicolson and Joanne Trautmann. New York: Harcourt Brace Jovanovich, 1975- 1980. Print.

_____. *Moments of Being.* New York: Harcourt, 1985. Print.

Wordsworth, William. *The Poems.* Vol. 1. Edited by John Hayden. New York: Penguin, 1990. Print.

Index